EATING YOUR WAY THROUGH LIFE

EATING
YOUR WAY THROUGH LIFE

JUDITH J. WURTMAN, Ph.D.

Research Associate
Department of Nutrition and Food Science
Massachusetts Institute of Technology
Cambridge, Massachusetts

Raven Press ▪ New York

Raven Press, 1140 Avenue of the Americas, New York, New York 100036

Made in the United States of America

Library of Congress Cataloging in Publication Data

Wurtman, Judith J
    Eating your way through life.

    Includes bibliographies and index.
    1. Nutrition. 2. Diet. I. Title.
RA784.W87   613.2   77-84128
ISBN 0-89004-280-2

To my husband Richard
whose love, wisdom, and wit
supported me throughout my writing

Preface

Several years ago I began to teach human nutrition at an undergraduate institution. Part of my preparation involved searching for a book that covered the subjects in the course: the nutrient needs and eating styles of people from infancy through old age, the use and safety of food additives, the benefits or hazards of megavitamins, the nutritional adequacy of alternate eating styles, the effect of dietary constituents such as cholesterol or fiber on health, the effectiveness of weight-reducing therapies, and methods of evaluating the nutritional adequacy of one's own diet. Although I found many books on nutrition, they were either traditional books for students in nutrition and dietetics, covered only one of these various topics, or dealt with rather nontraditional nutrition topics such as "garlic and long life" or "egg yolks and intelligence." The only solution seemed to be to write the book myself. Hence *Eating Your Way Through Life.*

My major objective was to develop methods of incorporating nutrient-rich foods into the eating styles of people of different ages that would satisfy their nutritional needs. I found myself thinking: How can a mother get her 2-year-old to eat the nutrients he needs if all he will eat is a small pancake, some apple juice, and two cookies? How can an 80-year-old woman get the calcium she needs if a quart of milk is too heavy for her to carry home from the market? How can a businessman who travels frequently meet his daily nutrient needs when he eats breakfast on an airplane and dinner at a business meeting?

I did not know many of the answers to these and other problems when I started to write. The answers came only after many hours of searching through food composition books, wandering through supermarkets, talking to people about the problems they had in obtaining the foods they knew they should be eating, and discussing my "solutions" with parents, social workers, teachers, friends, and students. I hope they are useful to the eaters reading the book.

Waban, Massachusetts

Acknowledgments

This book would not have been written without the constant support of my husband who supplied, in addition to encouragement, the title of the book. My children, Rachael and David, were also an enormous source of help and ideas, and were invaluable in collecting information about how their peers were eating.

I want to express my gratitude to Dr. Sanford Miller for reading and commenting on the book while it was in manuscript form and for his perceptive insights into the problems facing the American eater today. I also want to thank Mr. Joseph Carlin for his assistance and information on the nutritional needs of the elderly and Ms. Ruth Palombo for her review of my chapter on the nutritional needs of the adult. I want to thank Merriam Egan, Suzanne Fein, Louise Kittridge, and Christine Connaire for their help in editing and typing the manuscript and their comments on its contents. Finally, I wish to thank Dr. Diana Schneider for convincing me the book should be written.

Contents

A Look at the Past / Nutritient Needs of Childhood and Adolescence /
Eating Patterns During Childhood and Adolescence / References

Numbers / Nutrient Needs and the Problems Associated with Meeting
Them / Nutrition and Lifestyle of the Older Adult / Some Solutions /
Comment / References

Introduction

Most of us eat terribly, at least some of the time. We manage to go through a day, a weekend, or a week avoiding all of the food groups our teachers and mothers said were good for us. Some of us eat this way simply because we do not have the time to obtain and prepare certain foods, we want to restrict our calories, our financial restrictions limit our food choices, or the foods we should be eating are not available. Others of us eat this way because we really like "junk food," hate vegetables, cannot be bothered thinking about food, enjoy using up our calories on a hot fudge sundae rather than 2 pounds of cottage cheese, or would rather snack on what is handy than plan and prepare meals.

We are usually untouched by nutrition education campaigns, advertisements, and labels on the back of orange juice containers. Adding up our daily total intake of some obscure minerals or counting food groups is not compatible with our way of life. We give the nutritional aspects of our eating little if any attention.

Occasionally we are struck by the nutritional errors of our eating patterns. This usually happens after we have eaten Big Macs and french fries for 3 days in a row, or we cannot remember when we last drank some orange juice, or we walk past a health food store and feel unhealthy. Sometimes we try to compensate for these lapses in nutrient intake by a diet of vitamin pills, bone meal, and kelp. However, most of us quickly revert to our former eating style; the pills age, the bone meal is thrown on the garden, and the kelp is fed to the local goldfish.

Sometimes, however, we are no longer given the luxury of not caring about the nutritional quality of our diet. A doctor tells us we must start adhering to a particular diet because we are pregnant, fat, or have high blood pressure, cholesterol-filled blood, iron-poor blood cells, or sluggish intestines. Some of us may find ourselves responsible not only for the food we put into our own mouths but also into the mouths of others. Another eater appears in our lives—spouse, child, elderly parent, roommate—and meals must now have some rational nutrient content rather than the random nutritional value formerly characterizing them.

What is the eater to do? How does he change from a nutritionally apathetic eater into one with nutritional expertise and virtue? How does he manage to convince others to eat nutritionally well? This book offers guidelines, information, and suggestions to help in this transformation. The adult eater can learn how to change his eating style to incorporate nutritionally sound foods into his daily intake while keeping the structure of his personal pattern of eating intact. He can learn how to eat better even if faced with vending machines as his only source of lunch or the airlines as his source of dinner.

The busy, working, pregnant woman is advised on how to eat better nutritionally, as is the pregnant parent who tends to give her own food intake a low priority compared with that of her children. Parents are told how to contend with the eating styles of their toddlers, school-age children, and teenagers, and how covertly or overtly to improve their nutrient intake (even if the child thinks vegetables belong in the garden, not on the kitchen table). The developing eating style of the infant is also discussed, along with the pros and cons of breast-feeding, homemade or commercial baby food, and the basic nutrient needs of this rapidly growing person.

The eating styles of the older adult are discussed. The problems an elderly individual faces in purchasing and preparing food are considered as they directly affect his ability to satisfy nutrient needs. The individual who willingly, or because he has no choice, must reduce his food intake is also discussed.

The reasons for overeating are presented along with a detailed description of all the commonly available methods of weight reduction. The overeater is encouraged to choose a method of weight reduction compatible with his psychological and physiological needs.

Many eaters are not worried about the nutrients in their diets. They are more concerned about the nonnutritive substances they also consume, i.e., food additives and fillers. They find it hard to believe the assurances of the government that the additives are safe, yet are unwilling to accept the proclamations of doom by the natural food advocates who advise us to eat a chemical-free diet. (Since all food consists of chemicals, this is rather difficult to do.) People are also worried about the impact of certain foods on their health. They wonder whether they should avoid all eggs, eat only fiber and oranges, and allow themselves one salty anchovy a year. Some look to the nutrients that come in bottles rather than in food as the only reliable source of vitamins and minerals. They do not know if vitamin C is better for a cold than chicken soup, and whether the claims made for certain nutrients as therapeutic agents for wrinkles, baldness, and heart disease are true or simply wishful thinking. These issues are discussed and evaluated in the context of the most recent scientific information. Moreover, to enable the reader to keep up with changes in the status of some of these controversies, a list of recommended newsletters, pamphlets, monthly magazines, and journals which report on these areas is provided.

The book also helps the modern day hunter and gatherer of food make nutritious food choices and understand the complexities of food processing and labeling.

The influence of the American style of eating is discussed. Although the characteristic American eating style (fast foods, fast eating, convenience, vending machines) may not be representative of the way every reader of this book eats, it does influence the nutrient intake of many.

The function of the major nutrients in our diet is presented. However, since a chapter that contains nothing but paragraph after paragraph on the sources and functions of various nutrients makes somewhat dull reading, the function of the nutrients is described throughout the book in small doses. The index, however, guides the reader to this information, and the references provided enable him to read further if he wishes to acquire additional information.

1 THE AMERICAN WAY OF EATING

Judging from the array of foods available to the average American, it might be assumed that he spends most of his time eating or at least thinking about what to eat. He is rarely more than a short drive from an amazing variety of fast food restaurants, usually clustered near the outskirts of a town, where he can obtain hamburgers, tacos, hot dogs, whipped ice cream, and even a plastic-wrapped breakfast within a few seconds. He can enter any supermarket and choose among 10,000 to 12,000 items displayed in colorful clusters along the shelves. At work he usually has access to vending machines or snack bars, and at home he can find in his kitchen various boxes, cans, and pouches of food that require only minutes of preparation.

This variety and instant availability of food is characteristic of an American style of eating that has developed rapidly over the past 20 to 25 years. Several factors have contributed to the creation of this eating environment: new technology in food processing and distribution, innovative restaurant formats, and changes in the employment and recreation pattern of the American family.

Certain aspects of the American style of eating have been exported to other countries; for example, one can now buy McDonald's hamburgers in France, Germany, and Japan. However, many American inventions (e.g., frozen waffles, powdered breakfasts, and boxed hamburger "assistants") are still rare outside our borders.

In this chapter we examine the major aspects of the current, American way of eating, the factors responsible for its development and continuation, and the effect of this eating style on the nutritional quality of the American diet.

The environment in which we eat directly affects the way we interpret and use nutritional information. Theoretical nutritional requirements are irrelevant if they cannot be translated into the mode of eating followed by those for whom the requirements were developed. For example, lists of foods that contain specific vitamins or minerals are often used to help an individual select a diet that contains adequate amounts of these nutrients. However, unless the foods listed are familiar and easily obtainable, at home and in restaurants, they are eaten infrequently. For example, rutabagas are a good source of vitamin A, but how many people even recognize a rutabaga? If this turnip were to become a new item promoted by fast-food restaurants or advertised as the newest thing in snack foods, it might gain prominence as an important source of vitamin A. However, its place in the current American eating environment severely decreases its utility as a source of any vitamin or mineral because it simply is not eaten often enough.

Eating three nutritionally balanced meals a day is an objective with which we all agree but do not practice. If our life style causes us to skip breakfast and limit our lunch selection to the items offered by a nearby sandwich shop, we may not confront a "well-balanced" meal until dinner.

Elementary school teachers often use the four basic food groups as a guide for students in choosing food for each meal. However, for children whose parents follow a currently popular vegetarian diet, the "meat" and "milk" groups are completely meaningless.

These examples illustrate only a few ways in which our style of eating can affect the application and use of nutrition information. This chapter describes the current American *way* of eating, so that subsequent discussions on *what* Americans should be eating—i.e., their nutritional requirements—can be related to the context of the eating environment in the United States.

The American way of eating can be examined in terms of (a) the categories of foods available and (b) the factors motivating the acceptance or rejection of these foods. American foods can be classified as *efficient, healthy,* or *fun* foods, and each category brings with it a variety of reasons for acceptance or rejection in the American diet.

EFFICIENT FOODS

An efficient food can be defined functionally: It reduces the time between the desire to eat and eating. Efficient foods are termed "fast foods" when available in restaurants and "convenience foods" when prepared at home.

Fast Foods

Fast foods are served by a particular type of restaurant known as a fast-food chain. They are prepared under standardized conditions that utilize innovative technology to reduce preparation time and cost. The variety of such foods is relatively limited. A typical menu might offer a meat (hamburger or chicken), french fries, onion rings, and a soft drink, milk-based shake, or soft ice cream, and sometimes a filled tart misnamed "pie." Little variation appears in the menus of the national food chains, although local taste preference causes some small alterations in the food choices and ingredients used. For example, McDonald's hamburgers are prepared without mustard in New York City, coffee milkshakes are not available in Modesto, California, and fried chicken is currently being test-marketed in McDonald's franchises in the South.

The history of fast-food chains indicates that within relatively short time their orginal purpose—to serve food quickly to the automobile traveler—has been supplanted by a newer function: to offer an inexpensive fast meal of reliable quality to the urban employee and suburban dweller. New franchises are appearing in downtown business areas as well as suburban shopping centers. As the fastest growing segment of the away-from-home eating business (1), the fast-

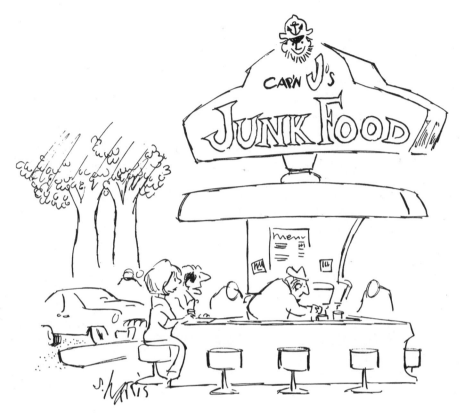

"Nice, unpretentious little place."

(Drawing by S. Harris; © 1976, The New Yorker Magazine, Inc.)

food franchise can be expected to affect the "eating out" habits of more and more Americans.

Recently a number of reports (1–3) have been published that compare the nutrient content of typical fast-food meals from several of the better-known franchises. These studies all reach similar conclusions—basically, that man cannot live by hamburgers, french fries, and milkshakes alone. He needs green leafy vegetables as well.

In addition, these reports showed that within the nutritional limitations of the fast-food menu, certain meal combinations offer more nutritional value than others. A study conducted by Chem and Lachance (1) demonstrated this finding by comparing the nutrient content of typical meals purchased from McDonald's, Kentucky Fried Chicken, Dairy Queen, and Burger King. The meal consisted of a hamburger, french fries, and a milk shake or soft drink from the hamburger chains, and chicken, coleslaw and potato, and a roll from the chicken chain. The food was analyzed for the following nutrients: protein, vitamin A, the B vitamins (thiamin, niacin, and riboflavin), vitamin C, calcium, and iron. Because standards for meal plannning suggest that each meal contain a third of the daily requirements of these and certain other nutrients, the nutritional value of the fast-food meals was evaluated on this basis.

All the food combinations tested had sufficient protein to meet standard requirements. However, several of the other nutrients tested varied in adequacy, depending on the food combination analyzed. The meals from the hamburger chains contained inadequate amounts of calcium, riboflavin, and niacin when a soft drink rather than a milk shake was the beverage. No meal combination met the requirements for thiamin and vitamins A and C due to the absence of fresh vegetables and fruits (suppliers of vitamins A and C) and inadequate enrichment of the rolls (a source of thiamin).

The chicken chain did even more poorly in this nutritional evaluation. A serving of Kentucky Fried Chicken, a roll, and coleslaw failed to meet the requirements for calcium, vitamin A, thiamin, riboflavin, and vitamin C; and if mashed potatoes were substituted for the coleslaw, the deficit in vitamins A and C and calcium was increased.

Should this analysis of the nutrient content of fast-food menus cause us to reach for a vitatmin pill? These nutritional deficiencies are real. However, the importance of these deficiencies to the nutritional health of the average American depends primarily on whether he relies on the foods served at these fast-food franchises to meet his daily nutritional needs. If this type of food represents the major food intake of the day, and if the food consumed during the rest of the day is chosen with little regard for its nutritional value, then the nutritional limitations of fast-food meals may affect nutritional health.

An occasional meal at a fast-food franchise should make the eater feel neither guilty nor malnourished. Even professional nutritionists do not consistently meet their nutrient requirements at every meal, and the amateur need not do so either.

Fast-food franchises comprise an important component of the American eating environment, and the ease and efficiency with which they provide food to the hungry American will support their continuation as an important aspect of the Amercan style of eating. It is almost as hard to imagine a highway today without the inevitable Golden Arches and Buckets of Chicken as to imagine it without an automobile, and one might expect both to have similar persistence in our way of life.

Convenience Foods

Convenience foods are to at-home meal preparation what fast foods are to away-from-home eating; both reduce the time between the desire to eat and eating. The proliferation of convenience foods into every aspect of home food preparation is astounding. The acceptance and use of such foods has had such a pervasive influence on home food preparation that someone preparing a dinner "from scratch"—i.e., raw materials—usually includes a large number of convenience food items without recognizing them as such. Salad dressings from bottles or powdered mixes, frozen vegetable combinations with special sauces, instant potatoes or rice, and a variety of boxed, pouched, canned, or frozen confections are commonplace in a meal "cooked" at home and displayed as representing a creation of the home chef. Were one to rid the kitchen of every food partially prepared for consumption before purchase, a dismayingly large number of food products would vanish from the refrigerator and cupboards.

Convenience foods are not uniquely American; occasionally a supposedly elegant and intricate French or Swiss food appears in its imported box or pouch in an American supermarket as instant souffle or fondue. However, American food technology has probably produced a greater array of convenience foods than its counterparts in other countries; and certainly American acceptance of, and reliance on, convenience foods makes them a dominant factor in our eating environment. Indeed a great deal of money and time are spent by marketing firms to detect gaps in the convenience product armament and to suggest products that will further reduce the time between preparing a meal and eating it. A casual survey of new convenience products described in a food industry trade journal (4) indicated that food preparation time will be shortened even further by the forthcoming addition to the supermarket shelves of such items as creamy potato bake, brown Italian cooking sauce, breaded frozen turkey sticks, and a two-toned, swirled frosting mix.

As a household increases its purchase and consumption of convenience foods, there is a concomitant decline in the number of foods prepared entirely in the home kitchen. When a category of convenience foods becomes accepted by the general public, rarely do the means of preparation revert to the methods used before the convenience food became available except for economic reasons. Extracting orange juice from the frozen juice container rather than from the orange is an example of an almost total switch from preparing a food item oneself to buying the finished product. The can opener is now the most efficient way to get orange juice on the breakfast table. In many households all cakes come from a mix, vegetables from a frozen box, and soup from a can, pouch, or cube.

Convenience foods are clearly taking over our kitchens. What effect does this phenomenon have on our nutritional well-being?

A definitive answer would require a long-term study comparing the nutritional intake of families eating food prepared entirely at home with that of other families who eat the same foods prepared and packaged commercially. Until such a study is done, we can only speculate on the effect of convenience foods on nutritional intake.

The nutritional consequences of eating convenience foods can be analyzed in another way, however, that may not be as scientific but which is more readily applicable to the individual's eating habits. The effect of convenience foods on nutrient intake can be evaluated by asking the following questions: (a) Would I eat the food if it were not already available in a convenient form? (b) Does the convenience food contain the same categories of ingredients and nutrients as it would if prepared at home?

The first question reflects the obvious but infrequently stated point that food does not nourish unless eaten. Certain foods (e.g., winter squash, dried beans) require so much preparation time—soaking, peeling, boiling, mashing, seasoning —that many people either avoid purchasing them or let them sit in the refrigerator or cabinet.

Uneaten, these foods obviously do not nourish. The same foods, already prepared for eating except for a final reheating, will be purchased and eaten. Convenience equals consumption in this case; and if they are nutritionally useful, the convenience foods can enhance the nutritional content of our diet.

To answer the second question requires label reading (also see Chapter 3, where the technology of food processing is discussed in some detail). However, if we follow the rewritten adage "You can't judge a frozen pizza by its picture on the box," then it may be possible to determine whether a convenience food has the same nutritional utility as the food prepared at home.

In the commercial preparation of various foods (e.g., pizza, fruit- or cream-filled pastry, chopped-meat dishes), certain ingredients we naturally associate with these foods (tomatoes, cheese, fruits, butter, cream, meat) are often replaced by less familiar ingredients (e.g., texturized starch, modified soy protein, or Torula yeast). When added to the appropriate juices (tomato, apple) or flavoring agents, texturized starch can mimic tomato paste, or fruit or cream pastry fillings. Soy protein or Torula yeast can be processed to replace a seemingly limitless variety of ingredients, including cheese and beef. Although these substitute ingredients have nutritional value, they are not the nutritional equivalent of tomatoes, cheese, eggs, or meat.

The nutrient density of a convenience food can also be altered by the addition of water or sugar. The food may have the same bulk or texture as the one prepared at home but, per mouthful, contain considerably fewer nutrients. Whether this difference in ingredient composition matters depends on the nutritional role the food plays in the daily dietary intake. For example, there is a frozen pudding that looks and tastes like the traditional pudding one makes by adding milk to a powder that comes in a box and heating the mixture until it thickens. Some prefer the frozen pudding because it tastes better, is not vulnerable to being scorched on the bottom, and is not covered with "skin." However, nutritionally it is far inferior to the add-milk-and-stir variety, as the milk content of the frozen pudding is much lower and the calorie content is higher.

Does choosing the prepared pudding over the one you fix at home have any nutritional consequences? If the frozen pudding is eaten for what it is—a tasty desert with minimal nutritional value—its nutrient content is irrelevant, as it has no nutritional function in the meal. However, if the pudding is served to fill the same nutritional purpose as the fixed-at-home pudding (which is to provide milk in an "eatable" form), then the nutritional content of the frozen pudding becomes important. Since the convenience pudding offers fewer nutrients per mouthful than the home-cooked pudding, eating the frozen dessert lessens the nutritional value of the meal.

Hence convenience foods can have a positive or a negative influence on nutritional status. When such foods entice us to eat a nutritionally valuable food, they are useful. When they appear as the nutritional equivalent of the cooked-at-home food but contain inferior ingredients, they decrease the value of our diets.

EFFICIENT FEEDING

If certain types of American foods are classified as "efficient," then the way many Americans eat can be described as "efficient feeding." Our desire to spend only a brief time eating meals has promoted our acceptance of and demand for foods that can not only be prepared rapidly but consumed quickly. Although our eating speed does not match that of a seal gulping his way through a bucket of fish, we often manage to eat our entire breakfast (such as it is) during the morning weather forecast or finish our vending-machine sandwich during the elevator ride back to the office. This decrease in the time Americans spend at meals, both at home and outside, and its resulting influence on the type of food we choose is related to our contemporary life style. Let us examine how the way we live affects the foods we choose to eat.

The Family Meal

Mealtime used to occur three times a day in the average American family. In the morning, at noon, and during the early evening members of the family gathered to eat a meal that usually consisted of several courses and that lasted at least an hour. Today we still find the American family coming together to share a meal: on Thanksgiving, at birthdays, and occasionally even during the week and on Sundays. However, the phenomenon of the family sitting down together three times a day is vanishing along with the napkin ring and the muffin warmer.

This shift from the daily meal-eating pattern to an irregular, individual-based eating schedule at home, as well as the increased consumption of food outside the home, has had an important influence on the American style of eating.

First, the elimination of specific time periods set aside for meals has resulted in an absolute decrease in the amount of time individuals spend in eating. This decrease in feeding time has directly affected the selection of foods eaten at those times of the day that were once set aside as mealtimes. The eating patterns exhibited by the typical American family at breakfast illustrate this point.

The current American breakfast demands foods that can be eaten rapidly, are movable (i.e., can be eaten away from the table or carried around the house), need only simple preparation, and appeal to the appetites of people who give early-morning eating a low priority. Another influence on the selection of breakfast food may be the necessity of preparing an item three or four times during a half-hour period as each member of the family becomes ready for breakfast. Preparation time may be limited even more if the person who prepares the meal must get ready to leave for work, car pooling, or school.

As a consequence of these stringent time requirements, traditional breakfast foods (homemade biscuits, muffins, bacon, omelets, hot cereal) have been replaced by convenience foods of the same name, or eliminated entirely. Instant breakfast drinks, cookies, and candy bars sold as nutritional equivalents to the traditional breakfast foods are increasingly accepted as they require minimal preparation and eating time.

The demands of the family's life style also affect the eating pattern throughout the rest of the day. The nature of the food choices, the presence or absence of meals, and the frequency of snacking are determined not by the family as a monolithic eating unit but by the specific needs of each member of the family. The requirement for an early dinner because of an after-supper ball game or for a later meal because of a 5:00 p.m. meeting may result in two dinners served on a particular day. If guests are invited for beef Wellington at 9:00 p.m., the children may dine on hot dogs at 6:00 p.m. School-age children, hungry when they arrive home because the school lunch was put in the trash, may eat their way through the afternoon and skip dinner entirely. Moreover, if several members of the family are absent at dinner time, whoever is eating at home may be served a cold sandwich or salad because "it is not worth cooking and cleaning pots for only one or two" (5). These examples indicate only a few ways in which the needs of the individual family member can influence the eating style of the entire family.

One component of the current American life style stands out as having a particularly significant impact on the eating habits of the American family: the growing number of women who are no longer at home during the day because of employment or other commitments outside the home. The "empty kitchen" resulting from the absence of the woman from the home is a relatively new phenomenon in the American family, but its effect on American eating habits has been so striking that the food industry considers it one of the most important factors in consumer buying habits.

In addition to claiming credit for freeing the woman from the kitchen (6), the large food corporations are now directing product development toward meeting the specific needs of the working wife and mother. Consequently, even more food items will probably become available in prepared or partially prepared form, and existing types of convenience foods will be modified to shorten further the preparation process.

Streamlining breakfast preparation is a major objective of the food industry, as it recognizes that the working wife/mother has a minimal amount of time to spend in the kitchen in the morning when she must leave the house with the rest of the family. Although products such as instant breakfasts are being advertised for their time-saving properties, some traditional convenience items (e.g., frozen orange juice) are now being regarded as obsolete by marketing analysts because they require too much toil and time. If these marketing analysts are correct, one can assume that the current American trend toward consumption of convenience food items will accelerate in the near future, and that they will represent an even larger proportion of the foods brought into the household.

The woman has traditionally been responsible for exerting some nutritional control over the food choices made by her family, and her absence from the kitchen necessarily affects not only the method of food preparation but also which foods are actually eaten. In the past, her influence on the nutritional quality of the family's diet ranged from the obvious (planning nutritious meals) to the subtle (tallying the intake of potato chips against vegetables and directing subsequent food choices to items with some nutritional value). Because she controlled to a large extent the foods available to the household through her choice of which foods to buy and serve at specific meals, she could respond quickly to the changing nutritional needs of her family. When certain members of the family were starting a diet, recovering from a cold, or temporarily following an irregular eating schedule because of the demands of a job, she was able to alter her food purchases accordingly. Although she was occasionally required to work like a short-order cook at a truck-stop, the wife/mother frequently managed to meet the shifting schedule of her family with something that resembled a meal.

The working wife/mother whose time in the home is limited will find it difficult to fulfill some of these functions, although with sufficient planning and delegating of responsibility she can to some extent continue to influence the eating patterns of the family. However, some nutritional "fallout" must result from the "empty kitchen," and it may take the form of careless food choices, overlooked nutritional needs, or inappropriate meal combinations. Whether this will have any effect on long-range nutritional status cannot yet be determined, as the exodus of women from the kitchen is too new. However, despite its newness, the influence of the working wife/mother on the American way of eating is already obvious.

Eating Away From Home

Eating away from home is another feature of the American style of eating that has gained importance in recent years. We all do it, from the 3-year-old eating snacks and lunch at nursery school to the senior citizen having his hot meal at the drop-in center. Fifty percent of all meals eaten by Americans last year were eaten away from home.

This figure may seem too high until one considers the variety of eating situations that occur outside the home. Most adults consume food in one or more of the following situations: coffee breaks (which often are surrogate breakfasts), lunches, afternoon snacks, and a hastily grabbed dinner at a fast-food franchise or a more leisurely consumed meal at a traditional restaurant; then, after the evening's recreation, there may be a snack to tide one over until breakfast. Some groups in the population eat all their meals away from home; these include persons living at school, camp, in the armed services, or in hospitals or convalescent or old-age homes.

Some of the food eaten at these meals is prepared at home and resembles, albeit more soggily, foods that might have been consumed at home. Many of these foods, however, are quite different from what would have been eaten at home and reflect not the individual's choice as much as the food selection available to him. Quite often individuals find themselves eating foods outside the home that they neither like nor prefer but eat anyway because the selection is limited. On an airplane, in a school lunch cafeteria, or at a vending machine lunchroom, the food choices are relatively small, and one either accedes to the choices available or goes hungry.

The variety of foods available in commercial eating establishments or institutional dining facilities is also sparse, and a predictable number and type of food items appear on the menus of these establishments. A lunch counter anywhere in the country offers the familiar menu of tuna, egg salad, hamburger, hot dog, or grilled-cheese sandwiches along with the daily special of chicken salad or crabmeat. School lunches listed in the local newspaper make dull reading, and corporation or institution cafeterias all seem to have liver on Thursday and baked fish on Friday.

Several factors contribute to this limited variety of foods. Centralized facilities prepare entrees and sell them frozen to restaurants and institutions, thereby reducing the cost of preparation compared with on-site cooking. An increasing number of restaurants are purchasing their food ready-made from such facilities. The result is that the variety of foods served by restaurants is limited since the types of precooked meals available are few. Several restaurants in the same area often serve similar foods—all purchased from the same centralized commissary. Eating facilities designed to feed a large number of people at a fixed cost tend to be conservative in their menu items, as they wish to minimize waste and decrease complaints. Items with limited appeal or familiarity usually do not appear in such facilities because the possibility of rejection is high. The armed services, camps, college food services, and airline catering firms are sensitive to the food preferences of the populations they serve and offer only those items that have the greatest acceptance and appeal. The effect of such criteria in selecting food results in a decrease in variety.

Another factor limiting the assortment of foods available when we eat out is the cost of preparing a large variety of items. This cost is probably the reason fast-food franchises have such restricted menus; the objective of this type of meal service is to prepare a high-volume item as inexpensively as possible.

People with specific nutritional needs are aware of the consequences associated with frequent reliance on food prepared away from home. One can usually identify those with special dietary needs by their backpacks full of lunch materials (boxes of cottage cheese, salt substitutes, low-fat crackers, tuna packed in water, and freezer containers full of chopped lettuce). Others who must subsist on fast foods, vending machine selections, or airline meals over long periods of time usually react with an irresistible longing for fresh vegetables or fruits.

Although it is not possible to identify precisely the nutritional deficiencies that may result from a complete, or at least frequent, dependence on restaurant food (there probably are none unless the meal selections are severely limited), one can speculate on what nutrients present in marginal amounts in the diet. Certain nutrients, such as the B vitamins, are not concentrated primarily in a few foods but are scattered in small quantities in a large variety of animal and plant foods. The ideal way to obtain the daily requirement of such nutrients is to eat an assortment of foods. Because many meals eaten away from home are repetitive and limited in variety (a doughnut for breakfast and a sandwich and soft drink for lunch), we may be obtaining only marginal amounts of certain nutrients. If a meal is skipped or thrown out, as is often the fate of school lunches, the nutritional deficit for that meal is total. One result of this pattern of eating has been to increase our reliance on the last meal of the day as the source of the nutrients we may have missed earlier. Hopefully, this meal contains the mix of foods missing from our earlier meals and compensates for any nutritional deficit. However, as we have already seen, eating at home has its own limitations.

The nutritional pitfalls associated with the American style of eating may cause one to give up on food as a source of nourishment. A happier conclusion is to increase the variety of foods eaten at home and away, even if this requires more time in selecting and preparing foods, or possibly lobbying in front of the local fast-food shop for rutabaga and salad on the menu.

FUN FOODS

A large number of the foods Americans eat can be described as "fun foods." These foods are enjoyable to eat or drink because of their taste and texture, and because they have pleasant associations. They are served as snacks at social gatherings or during leisure periods: occasionally they are eaten as a form of pleasant self-indulgence after a particularly unpleasant or frustrating task.

We crunch and chew our way through vast quantities of snacks and confectionaries and relieve our thirst with multicolored, flavored soft drinks, with and without calories, for two basic reasons. The first is simple: the food tastes good, and we enjoy the sensation of eating it. Second, we associate these foods, often without being aware of it, with the highly pleasurable experiences depicted in the advertisements used to promote their sale. Current television advertisements demonstrate this point: people turn from grumpiness to euphoria after crunching a corn chip. Others water ski into the sunset with their loved ones while drinking a popular soft drink. People entertain on the patio with friends, cook over campfires without mosquitoes, or go to carnivals with granddad munching away at the latest candy or snack food. The people portrayed in these scenarios are all healthy, vigorous, and good looking; one wonders how popular the food they convince us to eat would be if they would crunch or drink away while complaining about low back pain or clogged sinuses.

Other cultures also have their "fun foods." The English are "addicted" to chocolate, and one can identify an Israeli by the trail of sunflower seed husks he leaves. However, Americans outdo other cultures in the amount and variety of fun foods they eat; and, although they may be better off nutritionally without them and would certainly benefit calorically from their disappearance, it is hard to imagine the American eating environment without the sound of crunched potato chips or the metallic hiss of a soft-drink can being opened.

HEALTH FOODS

Does anyone eat food because of its nutritional value? The answer is yes, and the number of people whose eating choices are motivated by health and nutritional considerations is rapidly growing. A more detailed description of nutritionally motivated diets is given in Chapter 2. Let us concentrate here on how these people and the foods they eat (or avoid) have colored the American eating environment.

Just as we have labeled certain foods as fast, convenient, or fun, we have also gradually but noticeably classified particular foods as "health" foods. Many are still either confined to a store specializing in this type of merchandise or stuck in a corner of a supermarket on a health foods shelf. Certain items, unknown to the general public only a few years ago, are now displayed in general areas of the supermarket. Bean curd, wheat germ, soybeans, tigers milk cookies, spinach noodles, and other health foods may still be relatively unfamiliar, but they are being marketed nationally and are often purchased by someone who heard that they are "good for you."

Not too long ago the emphasis on, and demand for, "natural" foods (foods containing no artificial additives) by health food advocates and others was dismissed by the food industry as the grumbling of cranks. Today these same food manufacturers are adding a line of natural products to their more traditional ones and offer for national distribution many products formerly found only in health food stores.

Marketing analysts correctly predicted that "natural food" would become an important component of the American eating style. The food industry, following their advice, produced the natural products long before many of us could even spell granola.

Food advertising has changed as a result of this trend toward nutritious eating. It is not uncommon to find advertisements on television and in magazines extolling the virtues of a nutritious food or meal. Even advertisements directed toward children, long regarded by nutritionists as the wasteland of food advertising, are now showing their young viewers the necessity of eating well and are trying to convince them not to skip breakfast.

Generally, the effect of the health food movement has been to increase our awareness of the nutritional content of food, direct our food choices (to some extent to those items with some nutritional value), and perhaps make us feel guilty when we eat foods that taste good but provide only calories.

One aspect of the health food movement, however, may have a negative impact on our food choices. Certain foods are considered superior by the nutritionally motivated eater, and to those who have read books on the health food movement, dessicated liver, brewers' yeast, and honey come to mind. The practice of selecting foods with high nutrient density has led others who are somewhat familiar with the health food movement to refrain from eating any food without computing its nutrient content per mouthful. Foods that offer only one or two well-defined nutrients rather than half a dozen might not be eaten, even though the nutrients they provide meet our needs quite adequately for that specific vitamin or mineral.

Many foods are now being fortified with nutrients nature never intended them to contain in order to make them competitive nutritionally with health foods promoted by the nutritionally motivated eaters. Relying on such heavily fortified foods may deceive us into believing that a few such foods can provide all the nutrients required for that day. These foods are usually supplemented with 10 or so of the better known nutrients, and the consumer may not realize that he must obtain some 30-odd more nutrients to meet the daily requirements. Some of these nutrients are present in such small quantities they are called trace nutrients and rarely are added to foods during the fortification process. Since many are found in a wide variety of foods, it is assumed that they will inevitably be consumed along with the better known vitamins and minerals when the food is eaten. If we eat only foods containing the more familiar nutrients because they are added during the processing, we may not obtain some of the less known nutrients, which often are lost when foods are subjected to lengthy processing. None of us can afford nutritionally to limit our eating to the so-called nutritionally superior foods. Although it is true that certain foods are more compact nutritionally than others, none is without its nutritional limitations. Even the apple in the Garden of Eden had its drawbacks.

The American way of eating is constantly changing, and the trends outlined in this chapter may be replaced by others in the near future. Various subtrends reflecting geographic, ethnic, religious, or economic influences are also important in determining food choices in different parts of the country, neighborhoods, or even within families. Despite the vast amount of individual variation in food choices and the continuous adoption of new eating patterns, the factors affecting the American way of eating have probably influenced each of us. Although our response to these influences may vary, we can recognize something of ourselves in this description of the American eater.

REFERENCES

1. Chem, L-F., and Lachance, P. A. (1974): *Food Product Dev.,* 8:40.
2. Appledorf, H. (1974): *Food Technol.,* 28:50.
3. *Nutritional Analysis of Foods Served at McDonald's Restaurants.* University of Wisconsin Alumni Research Report. Madison, Wis., 1977.
4. Anonymous (1975): *Food Product Dev.,* 9:20.
5. Anonymous remark overheard at a Washington, D.C. playground, 1966.
6. Isserman, F. (1973): *Food Product Technol.,* 7:98.

2 THE IMPERFECT EATER: Eating During Adulthood

Many adults fail to eat a nutritionally complete diet every day, and some never eat such a diet any day. There are many reasons for this failure, but they all ultimately reflect the eating style of the adult and its influence on his food choices. The adult's eating style represents a composite of many influences: work, social and familial activities; geographic location; economic, ethnic, and religious status; his eating history with its myriad psychological associations; and his attitudes toward food as a status symbol, a symbol of celebrations and pleasant events, a source of good health, or therapy for sickness (chicken soup or vitamin C for a cold). Most importantly, his eating style represents his decided likes and aversions for certain foods. Eating to supply nutrients is often a minor consideration among these other influences on food choice.

> A professor actively engaged in nutritional research bumped into me in the vending machine area of our building. He was carrying his lunch just purchased from the machines: a small bag of peanuts, an icecream sandwich, and a cup of coffee. When I commented on the rather sparse nutritional value of these items, he laughed and said, "I eat what I like."

Although most of us "eat what we like," eating does have a purpose beyond the simple satisfaction of eating enjoyable foods. Food must supply us with the nutrients our bodies require. We cannot synthesize these nutrients and so we must rely on our food to provide them: vitamins, minerals, protein, essential fatty acids, and others. Fortunately, an enormous variety of foods is available in this country with which we can satisfy these nutritional needs. Unfortunately, an enormous variety of foods also exists which satisfies only our caloric needs (and sometimes even exceeds them). We often eat energy- or calorie-rich diets which are nutrient-poor.

Although the adult eater can "eat what he likes" and still perhaps manage to satisfy his nutritional needs, he is likely to be obtaining less than optimal amounts of some of the nutrients. To make sure he is eating a nutritionally adequate diet, he must pay some attention to its nutritional content. This does not mean that he can no longer "eat what he likes" or what is convenient, available, or affordable. He can continue to allow his personal eating style to be the major influence on his food choices. However, if his diet needs to be improved nutritionally, he should be willing to make small but important modifications in these food choices. How can he do this? First—by evaluating the nutritional adequacy of his diet. This chapter offers two methods for doing this. Second—by trying out and incorporating some of the suggestions in this chapter. These suggestions are designed to be integrated into a variety of eating styles and are practical, easy to follow, and involve foods likely to be eaten by the average eater. Suggestions for the vegetarian eater are also provided.

The adult eater is faced with another area of nutritional concern: the abundance of nutritional claims and controversies bombarding him from the media. He often is left confused and uncertain over what to eat and what effect his diet will have on his health, happiness, and longevity. It is difficult to pick and choose among the information as some of it is misleading, some valuable, and some contradictory or simply wrong. This chapter helps the eater evaluate this information.

MEETING THE NUTRIENT NEEDS OF THE ADULT

The nutrient needs of adults, known as the Recommended Dietary Allowances (RDA) (1) are based on the results of studies which established the amount of specific nutrients necessary to maintain normal functions in the body. These figures are applicable only to the healthy individual; they do not apply to people with acute or chronic illness, those who take medications that alter nutrient requirements, those who have genetically determined diseases that may alter their nutrient needs, or those who live under extreme climatic conditions. The nutrient needs for adults are listed in Table 1.

TABLE 1. Recommended daily intakes for adults

Parameter	Females		Males	
	Age 23–50	Age 51+	Age 23–50	Age 51+
Energy (Kcal)	2,000	1,800	2,700	2,400
Protein (g)	46	46	56	56
Vitamin A (IU)[a]	4,000	4,000	5,000	5,000
(RE)	800	800	1,000	1,000
Vitamin D	Satisfied by nondietary sources in adults. (If no source of sunlight is available, then a dietary source is recommended.)			
Vitamin E (IU)	12	12	15	15
Ascorbic Acid (mg)	70	70	70	70
Folacin (μg)	400	400	400	400
Niacin (mg)	13	12	18	16
Riboflavin (mg)	1.2	1.1	1.6	1.5
Thiamin (mg)	1.0	1.0	1.4	1.2
Vitamin B_6 (mg)	2.0	2.0	2.0	2.0
Vitamin B_{12} (μg)	3.0	3.0	3.0	3.0
Calcium (mg)	800	800	800	800
Phosphorus (mg)	800	800	800	800
Iodine (μg)	100	80	130	110
Iron (mg)	18	10	10	10
Magnesium (mg)	300	300	350	350
Zinc (mg)	15	15	15	15

From ref. 1.

[a]Retinol is the name of the preformed vitamin A which is found in animal foods. In plant foods vitamin A is found in the form of carotene. Carotene is converted by the body into retinol. One international unit of vitamin A is equivalent to 0.3 μg of retinol and 0.6 μg of β-carotene.

With the exception of calories, the nutrient values tend to exceed the requirements for most individuals. This is to ensure that those in the population whose needs might be slightly higher than those of the average individual will be covered by the recommendations. The National Academy of Sciences noted that "those who accept responsibility for estimating allowances tend to err on the positive side, for there is little evidence that *small* surpluses of nutrients are detrimental; deficits, even small ones, will, on the other hand, lead to deficiencies over the long period of time" [author's italics] (1). Most people satisfy their nutrient requirements if they eat 75% of the RDA for the adult.

The new edition of the RDA includes provisional allowances for nutrients omitted in previous editions. These nutrients include pantothenic acid, vitamin K, biotin, copper, manganese, fluorine, chromium, selenium, and molybdenum. The nutrient allowances are listed in Table 2. Descriptions of the function and food sources of these nutrients are found at the end of the chapter in the *Appendix*.

The exact requirements for some nutrients have not yet been established. These are minerals such as tin, vanadium, and nickel. No diseases associated with dietary deficiencies of these minerals have been found among humans; it is assumed that people who eat a relatively varied diet obtain enough of these minerals to satisfy their body's needs. However, their presence in unprocessed food and their absence in formulated or highly processed foods (liquid protein powders, powdered fruit drinks, soda, marshmallow fluff, soft ice cream, instant soups) are compelling arguments for eating a variety of relatively unprocessed foods daily. Vitamin and mineral supplements do not routinely contain these trace minerals. There are some supplements which do provide them, but since their actual requirements have not been established, relying on supplements is unwise. One can either obtain too much or ingest them in a form not efficiently absorbed or utilized by the body.

The nutrient requirements of the adult are loosely translated into a specific number of servings from the four basic food groups. They are listed in Table 3 and in Table 4 for vegetarians. (Although many nutritionists do not like to use the four basic food groups, there is no other model as simple as the basic four for telling us what we should be eating.) The number of foods in each group (and the list is

TABLE 2. *Provisional recommendations for trace element requirements*

Element	Amount (mg)
Copper	2.0–5.0
Manganese	2.5–5.0
Fluorine	1.5–4.0
Chromium	0.05–0.2
Selenium	0.05–0.2
Molybdenum	0.15–0.5

From ref. 1.
These requirements are made in terms of a range of values; further research will enable these nutrient requirements to be established more precisely.

TABLE 3. *What adults should eat daily*

I. Dairy products
- One or two servings
- One serving is the equivalent of:
  8 ounces milk
  1 cup cottage cheese
  1¼ ounces cheddar cheese or processed cheese
  1 cup yogurt
  1½ cup ice cream

II. Protein-rich foods (also known as the meat group)
- Two or more servings
- One serving is the equivalent of:
  2 to 3 ounces animal protein such as meat, poultry, fish, pork, lamb
  8 ounces beans, lentils, dry peas
  6 ounces soybean curd
  4 tablespoons peanut butter
  2 eggs
  3 ounces meat analogs (imitation meat products made from soybeans, nuts, or wheat)
  1½ ounces nuts (peanuts are not true nuts) or smaller amounts of several of these items)

III. Vegetables and fruits
- Four servings daily
- One serving is the equivalent of one piece of fruit (or vegetable if the vegetable is large like a stalk of broccoli) or ½ cup of the fruit or vegetable
- Include:
  One serving of citrus fruits or fruit juice or equivalent as ¾ cup green pepper, cabbage, strawberries, canteloupe, kale, tomatoes, Swiss chard, brussels sprouts, large baked potato

  One serving of spinach, romaine lettuce, escarole, broccoli, collard greens, beet greens, turnip greens, mustard greens, dandelion greens, butternut, Hubbard, or acorn squash, carrots, sweet potatoes, apricots, canteloupe, peaches, persimmons, watermelon, or pomegranate every other day

  One serving lettuce, peas, green or yellow beans, turnips, cucumber, eggplant, zucchini, pears, cherries, apples, blueberries, bananas, peaches, beets, or any other available fruit or vegetable not already listed

IV. Cereal-bread-grain products
- Four or more servings
- One serving is the equivalent of:
  1 slice bread, muffin, bagel, roll, bisquit, pancake, waffle
  1 ounce ready-to-eat cereal
  ½ to ¾ cup corn meal mush, grits, macaroni, noodles, rice, spaghetti, buckwheat groats, bulgur, wheat berries, barley, couscous, soy grits, or smaller amounts of several of these foods

V. Other
- 1 to 2 tablespoons margarine, cooking oil, butter
- Optional: about 1.5 ounces high-fiber food, unless it is eaten as part of groups III and IV

hardly exhaustive) indicates that an enormous variety of foods can be eaten that satisfy adult nutritional requirements. This is hardly surprising since man evolved and developed all over the world; consequently he either adapted to the foods available where he lived, or he died. Worms and steak, pigweed and broccoli,

TABLE 4. *What vegetarian adults should eat*

I. Dairy products
- One and a half to two servings
- One serving is the equivalent of:
  - 8 ounces milk
  - 1 cup cottage cheese or ricotta cheese
  - 1¼ ounces cheddar cheese, processed cheese, or other hard cheese
  - 1 cup yogurt
  - 1½ cup ice cream
- Nondairy eating vegetarians can obtain calcium by eating calcium-rich vegetables or soybean curd. About 2 cups broccoli; 1 cup collards, dandelion greens, watercress, kale, mustard greens, raw parsley; or 1 cup soybean curd contain approximately the same amount of calcium as 1 cup milk. Vitamin A can be obtained in these green vegetables as well as in yellow-orange ones like carrots; the vitamin D found in fortified dairy products can be obtained in cod-liver oil or by exposure to sunlight.

II. Eggs
- 1½ eggs (eggs can be used in quiches, souffles, custards, puddings, sauces, breads, mashed potatoes)
- Non-egg eating vegetarians should increase servings of group III

III. Protein-rich vegetable foods
- Two servings
- One serving is the equivalent of: 1 cup cooked soybeans, chickpeas, lentils, pinto, kidney, navy beans,
  - ¼ cup peanuts or peanut butter
  - 6 ounces soybean curd
  - 3 ounces meat analogs made from soy, nut, or wheat protein
  - 1½ ounces or 3 tbs cashews, cashew butter, walnuts, pecans, pistachios, or sunflower, pumpkin, squash, or sesame seeds
- Nondairy or egg-eating vegetarians should eat three servings from this group

IV. Cereal-bread-grain products
- Males: eight servings
- Females: six servings
- One serving is the equivalent of:
  - 1 slice whole grain bread, ⅓ or ½ cup granola-type cereal, ¾ cup cooked whole grain or enriched cereal
  - 1 cup cold whole grain or enriched cereal
  - ¾ cup cooked, enriched whole grain or soy macaroni, noodles, spaghetti
  - 1 biscuit, muffin, pancake, bagel, waffle
  - 1 tbs wheat germ
  - ¾ cup cooked brown, converted, or enriched rice
  - ¾ cup bulgur, kasha, soy grits, wheat berries
  - 1 large cookie made with whole-grain-like oatmeal

V. Fruits and vegetables
- Males: six servings
- Females: five servings
- One serving is the equivalent of ½ cup or one piece of fruit (or vegetable if it is large like a stalk of broccoli)
- Include: one serving of citrus fruits or fruit juice or equivalent as:

  ¾ cup green pepper, cabbage, strawberries, canteloupe, kale, tomatoes, Swiss Chard, brussels sprouts, large baked potato

  One serving spinach, romaine lettuce, escarole, broccoli, collard greens, beet greens, turnip greens, mustard greens, dandelion greens, butternut, Hubbard, or acorn squash, carrots, sweet potatoes, apricots, canteloupe, peaches, persimmons, watermelon, or pomegranate

(contd.)

TABLE 4 (contd.)

One serving lettuce, peas, green or yellow beans, turnips, bean sprouts, pears, plums, beets, cucumber, eggplant, zucchini, pears, cherries, apples, blueberries, bananas, grapes, or any other available fruit or vegetable

---

Adapted from ref. 52.

jellied calves feet, and milk supply similar nutrients (protein, vitamin A, and calcium, respectively); only their culinary appeal differs. It is also obvious from looking at the four food groups chart that diets which are severely limited in variety are deficient in nutrients regardless of whether they consist of soda and french fries or soy milk and alfalfa sprouts.

Although every food group provides a variety of nutrients to the diet, each group is an especially good source of specific nutrients. This is the basis for the number of servings recommended from each group and should be the basis on which the foods from each group are selected. For example, one can meet the vegetables and fruit group requirements by eating celery, cucumbers, and radishes or by eating citrus fruits, carrots or spinach, and cucumbers. The first choice of vegetables provides little except water and fiber to the diet; the second provides vitamins and minerals in addition.

Dairy Group

The dairy group is an excellent source of calcium. Although certain vegetables (e.g., kale, collard greens, mustard, dandelion, turnip, beet greens) also supply calcium, these vegetables are included less frequently (an understatement) in a meal than dairy products. Thus we have come to rely on milk, yogurt, cottage cheese, hard cheeses, ricotta cheese, and even ice cream as a source of this important mineral. Most dairy products contain (or are fortified with) vitamin A. Milk is fortified also with vitamin D. Dairy products are a good source of protein, riboflavin, and a relatively good source of zinc.

Meat Group

The meat group (this is a misnomer since nonmeat products are included) is the major source of protein in the diet. Three ounces of meat (i.e., the size of a MacDonald's hamburger) supplies 20 to 25 grams of protein, which is about half of the amount required daily. Proteins are made up of amino acids and are therefore a source of the amino acids the body cannot make itself (the essential amino acids) as well as those synthesized by the body (nonessential amino acids). The best sources of essential amino acids are animal protein (meat, poultry, eggs, fish, dairy products) since their essential amino acid content meets the needs of our bodies. Plant protein contains considerably smaller amounts of some of the essential amino acids we need; fortunately not all plant proteins are deficient in the same essential amino acids. Legumes such as kidney beans, lima beans, and black-eyed peas, and grains such as rice, corn, and buckwheat groats lack different essential amino acids. If eaten together, these two plant foods (legumes and grains) complement each other's deficiencies. This is also true of nuts and seeds, which supply amino acids missing in legumes and grains. Books such as *Diet for a Small Planet* (10) and others on vegetarian cooking offer recipes for combining complementary plant proteins. A list of supplementary reading on vegetarian diets is provided at the end of the chapter. It is possible of course to reduce one's consumption of meat without becoming a true vegetarian. Many people are doing this today in order to reduce their intake of saturated fat. An easy way to accomplish this is to switch from high-fat meats such as beef, pork, and ham to lower-fat-containing meats such as chicken (without the skin), fish, and lean beef. Another is to follow recipes for vegetarian dishes and add small amounts of meat for flavoring.

In addition to supplying protein, the meat group provides zinc, riboflavin, iron, thiamin, vitamin B_{12}, potassium, and chromium; liver supplies all these plus vitamin A and folic acid.

Vegetable and Fruit Groups

Two subgroups of fruits and vegetables are singled out for daily or frequent consumption because they provide a variety of nutrients. The citrus fruit group is an excellent source of vitamin C; small quantities supply the daily requirement, or larger quantities of other vitamin C-containing fruits and vegetables can be substituted. Such alternates include strawberries, green pepper, baked potato, cabbage (raw or cooked in a small amount of water), "greens," raw spinach, broccoli, watermelon, and canteloupe.

Dark-green leafy vegetables are superb suppliers of vitamins A and C, folic acid, calcium, potassium, and even iron (although iron is not as well absorbed from plant as from animal sources such as meat). These leafy vegetables also contain few calories. They have only one disadvantage: Few people eat them.

Yellow-orange fruits and vegetables are an excellent source of vitamin A. A word of caution, however: The skin of people who consume vast quantities of these foods has been known to develop a yellow-orange hue.

The enormous category of "other" vegetables and fruits supply smaller quantities of vitamins A, C, and B_6, folic acid, potassium, magnesium, and manganese. Moreover, most vegetables and fruits are good sources of fiber, primarily in the form of pectin.

Bread–Cereal–Grain Group

Foods from the bread–cereal–grain group have a higher concentration of nutrients when they are less processed. Wheat germ is one of the least processed components of wheat and is an excellent source of zinc, folic acid, vitamin B_6, thiamin, riboflavin, niacin, vitamin E, and a variety of trace minerals such as chromium, manganese, cobalt, copper, selenium, and molybdenum. Each of these nutrients is found in lesser amounts in other grain products; more of course is found in whole wheat than in white flour goods, and in brown rice than in instant white rice. Certain grain products (e.g., breads, cereals, pastas) are enriched with some of the nutrients lost during processing; however, except for iron, trace minerals which are lost are not usually replaced by mineral fortification. Some of the foods in this group (e.g., bran or whole wheat flour) are good sources of fiber.

It is important to read the labels on bread or cracker products to determine if they contain whole grain flour or bran. The dark color of bread or crackers may be due to caramel coloring, not whole wheat flour.

VEGETARIAN DIET

The vegetarian can obtain the recommended amounts of nutrients easily if he includes dairy products and eggs in his diet. Table 4 shows the recommended number of servings from various food groups for the vegetarian eater. Eliminating dairy products omits a valuable source of calcium from the diet, but calcium can be obtained in dark green leafy vegetables and soybean curd (tofu). Vitamin B_{12} is also scarce in a diet lacking dairy products and eggs; some types of seaweed are thought to provide this nutrient, but it might be wise for the strict vegetarian to check with his physician about vitamin B_{12} supplements if his diet contains no animal products (the major source of this vitamin). Although sunshine provides vitamin D, vegetarian eaters who live in a cloudy, rainy, snowy, or cold climate should consider adding vitamin D to their diet in the form of fish oil or supplements (be careful, however, in the amount of supplement used; vitamin D toxicity results from large intakes). The list of references on vegetarian eating provides more detailed information about nutrient requirements and how they can be met.

Vegetarian eaters now can buy "convenience" foods. They are sold in health food stores and consist of vegetarian meals in a reheatable pouch. An example is fruit and nut rice, which consists of brown rice, raisins, sunflower seeds, sesame seeds, raw peanuts, and a special spice blend. It cooks in 45 to 50 minutes. Another is mushroom-wheat pilaf, which contains bulgur wheat, mushrooms, onions, and a special vegetable blend of soybeans, carrots, peas, spinach, parsley, celery, and a natural herb seasoning. It cooks in 20 minutes.

Many types of meat analogs are also available for the vegetarian. These products are made from soy protein and resemble meat or chicken dishes in appearance and flavor. Examples include vegetarian "hamburgers," "hot dogs," "steak," "cutlets," "bacon," and "sausage." These products are available in health food stores and come canned or frozen. Some (e.g., vegetable sausages, bacon, and ham slices) are available frozen in supermarkets.

MACROBIOTIC DIET

The macrobiotic diet is gaining in popularity in urban areas in the country. Although no animal product is included in this diet, it bears only a superficial resemblance to the vegetarian diet. Food choice for the macrobiotic is determined by ideological considerations rather than health or nutritional considerations. There are seven possible diets to follow. Each succeeding diet is more limited in food choice, and the final diet consists primarily of brown rice. An example of the most flexible diet, stage 1, is shown in Table 5. Foods are thought to possess certain qualities (heat or cold, sweetness or saltiness, roughness or smoothness, dryness or wetness, softness or brittleness). Each meal must consist of foods which balance these qualities. Moreover, each meal must contain a certain amount of brown rice, vegetables, salty condiments, seaweed, and legumes. The types of vegetables, beans, and condiments allowed vary with the season of the year and geographic location.

The difference between the vegetarian and macrobiotic diets is shown in Table 5.

Certain nutrients may be difficult to obtain in sufficient quantities on a strict macrobiotic diet: vitamins D, B_2, and B_{12}, and zinc, calcium, and iron. Fortunately, some traditional macrobiotic foods are good sources of these nutrients.

Miso, a fermented soybean product that often contains wheat, barley, or rice, is a good source of protein, several of the B vitamins including B_{12} (made by the yeast and bacteria used for the fermentation), and calcium. Tofu or soybean curd is a good source of protein, B vitamins, and calcium. Brown rice, buckwheat groats, soy grits, millet, rye, barley, beans, and lentils, which comprise a substantial part of the macrobiotic meal, are good sources of the B vitamins and several minerals (e.g., chromium, magnesium, manganese, iron, and molybdenum).

TABLE 5. *Daily food intake of a macrobiotic (stage 1) and a vegetarian eater*

MACROBIOTIC DIET

Morning	*Afternoon*	*Evening*
3 pieces wheat gluten	1 maple walnut cookie	1 cup brown rice
2 tsp aduki beans	3 tbs aduki beans	1 cup hiziki seaweed
1 "bite" kombu seaweed	¼ cup onion, carrots,	sauce for rice: parsley,
5 cups Bancha tea	broccoli	carrot, onion, uneboshi
¼ cup raisins	1 cup fried brown rice	plum, tahini
1 cup miso soup	and millet	⅓ cup aduki beans
		½ cup yams

VEGETARIAN DIET

Morning	*Afternoon*	*Evening*
1 cup whole wheat cereal	1 cup black beans	2 cups vegetable soup
1 tbs raisins	and rice	¾ cup cooked collard
1 tbs molasses	½ cup coleslaw	greens
1 slice whole wheat toast	1 banana	whole wheat bread
1 orange	2 slices date bread	corn on the cob
1 tbs peanut butter	small salad: lettuce and	margarine
	tomato with salad	½ cup cashew nuts
	dressing	soybean "meat" loaf (1 slice)

Carrots are an important source of vitamin A; dark green leafy vegetables provide vitamin A, folic acid, and calcium. Seaweed supplies essential amino acids in concentrations similar to those found in such animal proteins as milk or meat. It also contains iron, many trace minerals, and possibly vitamin B_{12}.

Vitamin D is very difficult to obtain in the macrobiotic diet, and parents are advised to give their children codliver oil to prevent rickets. A good source of information on the nutritional value of macrobiotic food was recently published (11).

DETERMINING NUTRITIONAL INTAKE

In order to eat better nutritionally, it is necessary to learn what one is actually eating. We all have notoriously poor memories of our food intake; we underestimate our calories and overestimate the nutritional value of our food choices, and we usually forget most items eaten standing up, in the car, or before going to bed. The only way to learn what you actually eat every day is to write everything down.

Ideally a food record should be kept for an entire week or 10 days scattered over a 2- to 3-week period. However, since other needs compete for the same time, try to keep a food record for at least 3 or 4 days. If these days are typical eating periods (i.e., they do not coincide with a period of intense dieting, work- or family-related stress, sickness, vacation, or being confined to the house during a blizzard), the food record should show you what you normally eat.

The following is a simple method for keeping a food record.

1. Use a small looseleaf notebook. Date the pages so they can be removed and carried individually if the notebook is too bulky to fit into a pocket or purse. After the pages have been filled in, put them back in the notebook in chronological order.

2. Record all food and beverages consumed. If you measure the quantity and size of portions at home, you can then estimate portion sizes when you eat away from home. It is not necessary to be exact about quantity; however, you should know whether you are drinking 4 or 5 ounces of orange juice, for example, or 10 to 12 ounces.

3. Try to be "typical" in your food choices on the days you are keeping a record. There is no prize for the best or worst food intake. Eating only nutritionally valuable foods on the days you write down what you eat prevents you from learning whether there are normally some nutritional "gaps" in your diet.

4. Write down where the food was eaten and its source: home, restaurant, vending machine, sidewalk pushcart, airplane, candy counter, car, party, and so forth.

5. Note the times of day when you eat.

After a food record has been kept for several days, its nutritional adequacy should be evaluated.

1. Roughly group the foods into the four food groups. Since this is difficult with certain food combinations like pizza or a "Big Mac," try to determine the major

ingredients in these combination dishes and place them in appropriate groups. The pizza, for example, contributes to the bread group, the vegetable and fruit group (tomato sauce), and the dairy group (cheese).

2. Compare the number of servings of each food group met by your food intake each day with the recommended number. Note in particular whether the foods you ate from each group were relatively good or poor sources of the nutrients each group is supposed to supply. For example, did you satisfy the dairy group requirement with milk or ice cream, the bread group with brownies or bran flakes, the vegetable and fruit group with cucumber or oranges, and the meat group with bacon or liver? The chart in Table 3 lists nutritionally valuable members of each food group.

3. Look for an insufficient number of servings or actual omissions from the food groups. If they occur day after day, note this. However, be flexible in interpreting this part of the food record. Sometimes you will compensate for an omission from a food group on one day by eating several extra servings on another day. Focus primarily on repeated rather than random omissions. For example, you may find that you never drink milk on weekends but that you eat yogurt for lunch and drink milk with supper every day during the week. Clearly you are then obtaining sufficient food from the dairy group. Conversely, you may find that you eat no foods which supply vitamin C; you do not drink citrus fruit juice and never eat any of the other items that supply this vitamin. This is an important omission and should be corrected.

Analyzing the nutritional quality of one's diet by using the four food groups is useful and does not require much time. It does not, however, give an exact accounting of the nutrient content of the diet as the foods which satisfy the serving number of each food group vary in their nutritional content. To learn what the nutrient content of one's daily intake is and how it differs from the nutrient requirements set forth in the RDA, it is necessary to do a nutrient analysis of the foods one eats. For those who are interested in doing so, Table 6 outlines the method.

As mentioned earlier in the chapter, eating less than 75% of the RDA indicates that one's nutrient requirements are not being met (unless one is obtaining the nutrients in vitamin or mineral supplements). However, certain nutrients do not have to be eaten every day; obtaining them a few times each week is sufficient. These are the fat-soluble vitamins—A, D, E, and K (the latter is made in substantial amounts by gut bacteria)—which are stored in the body. Calcium, phophorus, zinc, and iron are also stored in the body and are thus available when none is supplied by the diet. Most people who regularly consume an adequate amount of nutrients can eat very little of nutritional value for a few days and suffer few ill effects. Indeed we all do this many times, such as during a short illness, when traveling, during a snowstorm, when the electricity fails, or during a spell of hot weather when the appetite decreases. However, a chronic insufficiency of any nutrient leads eventually to the body's stores being used up.

TABLE 6. *How to calculate daily nutrient content*

---

1. Write down all the food eaten on a given day. Record its weight, size, or volume.
    a. It will be necessary to measure the foods. Use a food scale, measuring cup, or tape measure. Some items will have to be estimated: a small banana, a medium-sized apple.

2. If a food contains several ingredients, try to estimate the relative amount of each. For example, a cup of stew may contain 3 pieces of meat, ½ cup carrots, ¼ cup gravy, ⅛ cup potato.

3. Use a food composition book to look up the nutrient content of the food.[a] (Some nutrients such as trace minerals, vitamins B_6, and B_{12}, and folic acid are not listed; however, these nutrients are found in association with many of the nutrients listed.)
    a. The simplest nutrient analysis of food involves tabulating its content of the following nutrients: vitamins A and C, thiamin, riboflavin, calcium, magnesium, and iron. Others may be included along with the caloric, fat, protein, and carbohydrate content of the foods.
    b. If the amount of food eaten is larger or smaller than the amount listed in the table, increase or decrease its nutrient content accordingly.

4. Add up the total amount of each nutrient consumed on a given day. To compare this figure with the amount that meets RDA standards, divide the daily amount of the nutrient consumed by the recommended amount and multiply by 100. This gives the percent of the RDA contributed by the diet on a given day. For example, if the daily total calcium intake was 400 mg, it represents 50% of the RDA for adults $(400 \div 800 \times 100 = 50\%)$.

---

[a]Two food composition books are listed under *Recommended Reading* at the end of the chapter.

After learning about one's nutritional intake, the food record should be scrutinized to learn about one's eating style. Note the types of foods usually eaten, which ones are avoided or eaten infrequently; where eating takes place; how often and when nonnutritive food is eaten; the types of meal eaten or skipped; and the times during which one has control over what is eaten and when the decision is left to someone or something else (e.g., what is left in the vending machine at 2 p.m. or the content of the lunchtime special). This information can be used to make nutritionally beneficial adjustments in food intake. The following are examples of how this can be done.

IMPROVING NUTRITIONAL INTAKE

Morning Meals

Use the morning eating periods (breakfast or coffee break) to choose foods from the dairy, citrus fruit, and grain groups. Nonbreakfast eaters can modify their eating habits slightly to include a citrus fruit or juice, a cup of coffee or tea with milk, and perhaps a piece of whole wheat toast. If this meal is ignored, orange or grapefruit juice and a half pint of milk can be substituted at the coffee break along with the cup of coffee and danish. With some foresight, a small box of cereal or raisins or a banana or orange could be carried to work to munch on during this midmorning eating. If pastries or bread products are eaten at this time, try to make them a bran muffin or whole wheat bread; these foods contain fiber and several vitamins and minerals that are absent from doughnuts, pastries, or white flour-based muffins and rolls.

Lunch

If you eat away from home, try to eat whole grain rather than white bread; ask for lettuce and tomato on sandwiches; drink milk or fruit juice instead of soda; and buy fruit or yogurt with fruit for dessert, or bring an apple, banana, or orange from home.

If you commonly eat at full-service restaurants, consider ordering the following foods: baked potato rather than french fries or potatoes in sauce, a salad, cooked vegetables (especially dark green leafy ones, such as spinach, or yellow-orange ones, such as carrots or squash), fish instead of meat (it has a lower fat content), liver (if iron-rich foods tend to be low in your diet), shellfish (they are excellent sources of zinc, copper, magnesium), and fruit and cheese for dessert if you eat dessert. Should the caloric content of a restaurant meal be a problem, order milk rather than cream for coffee or tea, oil and vinegar instead of a salad dressing; avoid or consume few alcoholic drinks, and rolls and butter. Instead of a calorie-laden appetizer, order broth, fruit juice, or half a grapefruit. Ordering a salad as soon as you sit down prevents you from filling up on bread and butter.

Vending machine dining poses problems if the machines are out of foods that have nutrient value by 10:00 a.m. Go to the machines when you come to work, buy your lunch, and store perishables in an insulated "beach bag" under your desk. Select sandwiches, hot soup, stew, pasta in cans, fruit, yogurt, and (if available) eggs, pizza, or pancakes. If the machines are out of entree items, you can still get milk, juice, raisins, peanuts, packaged granola, or even ice cream; at least these foods provide some nutrients with their calories.

At fast food franchises, watch calories because a considerable amount can be consumed in the form of milkshakes, french fries, fruit pies, soda, and extra layers of bread, mayonnaise, or tartar sauce (12). Order milk not milkshakes, unadorned rather than layered hamburgers or cheeseburgers (you do not need the extra bread and sauce), and hold the french fries and apple pie—look for fruit on the way back to work.

If lunchtime is also errand time, pack some portable foods that can be munched. This reduces the temptation to buy an ice cream cone or a doughnut and coffee. Bananas, carrots, a green pepper, small packages of seeds, dried fruit, or nuts (unless calories are a problem), a small wedge of cheese, chunks of red cabbage, and whole wheat crackers make nutritionally respectable snacks.

Midafternoon and Before-Dinner Snacks

If the food intake record indicates that many calories but few nutrients are consumed late in the afternoon or as before-dinner appetizers, anticipate this hungry period and stock the office, car, briefcase, pocketbook, and refrigerator with nutritious but relatively low calorie foods. You must plan ahead to be successful in this. Save a muffin from breakfast, a fruit from lunch, or even cold vegetables from the night before (the latter can be marinated—pour some salad dressing over them—and eaten as a cold vegetable appetizer). Have cut raw vegetables, such as green pepper, carrots, cucumber (or a pickle), or a hardboiled egg in your car or briefcase to reach for, rather than a candy bar, on the way home from work. Eat some food from the dairy, grain, or vegetable group as a substantial snack before dinner if this is a time in which large doses of potato chips or corn chips are usually consumed. Soup containing vegetables, chickpeas, noodles and even small pieces of bean curd can be eaten as a nutritious and filling first course or appetizer and satisfies several of the food group requirements. Dip raw vegetables in seasoned yogurt or munch on some sunflower or sesame seeds (these are extremely good sources of several nutrients for those who can afford the calories) or have some seasoned cottage cheese or hard cheese on whole wheat crackers or whole wheat toast.

Dinner

In order to fill the daily grain and vegetable–fruit requirements, include as many unprocessed or slightly processed foods as possible in the dinner meal. It takes no more time to prepare such grains as rice, kasha, pasta products, or barley than it does to read the directions and prepare a box of highly processed rice, noodles, or pasta. Stay away from side dishes such as stuffing mixes if they represent your major source of grains for the day. The major component of these stuffing products is flour, and they lack the vitamins and minerals present in whole grain products. Kidney beans, peas, lima beans, or chickpeas take more time to prepare if they are raw; however, these all come in cans and can be added to a variety of dishes from stews to soup, salads, or rice casseroles. They can also be used to thicken gravies if blended or mashed first. Steaming vegetables is the fastest and least fussy way of preparing them, and the vegetables retain their nutrients and crispness. Steaming is useful for preparing frozen as well as fresh vegetables, and it takes no more time than preparing a salad.

If you see from your food record that your food intake is repetitious and limited in variety, you may not be getting sufficient amounts of all the nutrients you need. Try to eat some new types of grains, vegetables, or legumes. However, do not experiment with these unfamiliar foods when you are rushed. Buy the novel foods, store them, and experiment with different ways of preparing them on weekends, snow days, or holidays. Try these new foods in frozen or canned form first if you are not sure how to prepare them. Most vegetables are available in frozen form and some come seasoned or with sauces. Many dried beans are also available in cans (chickpeas, kidney beans, baked beans), and some of the whole grains (e.g., brown rice) have been processed so they do not turn sticky after cooking. Another way of trying these foods is in a restaurant. For example, restaurants serving Middle Eastern cuisine often have bulgur or chickpeas on the menu.

Dinner should be used as a time to eat foods that are difficult to obtain at other meals and also to compensate for nutritional gaps. Drink fruit juice or milk if these foods were absent from earlier meals; eat yogurt, fruit, or both for dessert to satisfy dairy group and vegetable–fruit group needs; and include some whole grain foods if possible. (Wheat germ on ice cream makes a nice dessert.)

After-Dinner Munching

Some people eat most of the total daily food intake between 6 and 11 p.m. Unfortunately they rarely eat kale, lima beans, liver, or grapefruit. The food intake record is useful for helping the nocturnal eater gain nutrients (rather than weight). If you like to eat at night, plan the snacks and mini-meals so they make nutritional sense. For example, you could eat breakfast late in the evening, thereby saving time in the morning as well as meeting nutrient requirements. If fiber consumption is low during the day because most of the food was highly processed, eating a bowl of bran (and milk), a bran muffin, a dish of coleslaw, several carrots, or some baked potato skins (saved from supper) would quickly increase your fiber intake to healthy levels. Snacking on seeds, nuts, raisins, figs, or apricots rather than pretzels and popcorn adds immeasurably to your nutrient intake. Since more time is usually available in the evening to plan, prepare, and consume food, make the food choices meet your nutritional needs. When planning these snacks, incorporate foods which are overlooked or avoided earlier in the day.

At-Home Eaters

Those who do most of their eating at home are at both an advantage and a disadvantage. They have access to whatever they want to eat when they want to eat it. Easy access, however, makes it possible to eat too many calories, and if they are casual about the nutritional value of their food choices they can eat too few nutrients. The following suggestions may help solve these problems.

1. Buy only foods which have some nutritional value; leave the cookies, potato chips, soda, crackers made with unenriched flour, and cupcakes on the super-market shelves. Fill the kitchen with nutritional munchables such as carrots, bananas, yogurt, cereal, whole grain bread and crackers, seeds, dried fruit, canned fish, cheese, cottage cheese, and eggs. Then, when "appetite strikes," you will eat something that is nutritious since there is nothing else available.

2. Keep a careful food record. Leftovers count but are usually overlooked, especially when they consist of a 2-year-old's lunch or the remains of the family breakfast. Do not feel it necessary to eat what others do not want; plan your meals around your own nutrient needs and make sure they include nutritionally valuable foods from the four food groups (see Table 2 and text for examples).

3. Keep a large bowl of cooked or raw vegetables in the refrigerator, some bran muffins on the counter, and soup, tunafish, and whole wheat bread in the cupboard so the components of a meal are available. This decreases the temptation to grab something less nutritious at meals.

The Single or Small-Household Eater

Some eaters have little or no interest in the selection or preparation of food, and they consider eating—and even worse, eating for nutrient content—to be unworthy of their attention. These people are apt to be one of the growing subgroup in the population who live in single or small households; a recent survey predicts that they will comprise about 55% of the population by 1980 (13).

The life style of this subgroup clearly influences their food choices. Foods are selected that require little time and work to prepare and even less to clean up. Perishable foods or large serving sizes are avoided so an impulsive decision to go away for a weekend does not result in a refrigerator filled with sour milk or moldy leftovers. A good deal of the eating occurs outside the home, and food selection at home tends to be repetitious and simple.

A solitary eater is apt to make food choices that are deficient in the vegetable–fruit and dairy groups, and in whole grain products. Most of the carbohydrate consumed is likely to be in the form of hamburger buns, potato chips, and doughnuts.

The nutrient intake of such an eater improves only if he can easily change his food choices so they remain compatible with his eating style and lack of interest in his nutritional state. Some suggestions to this end are as follows:

1. Stock the kitchen with relatively nonperishable but highly nutritious items so eating at home provides some of the nutrients apt to be missing in the diet of a chronic restaurant eater. Wheat germ is an excellent source of vitamin B_6, folic acid, vitamin E, zinc, thiamin, riboflavin, and magnesium, as well as several other minerals. One or two tablespoons in yogurt, applesauce, ice cream, or pancake mix or added to cereal can compensate for possible nutritional gaps in the day's food choice.

2. Carrots, oranges, bananas, grapefruit, and green pepper can be stored for a few weeks at least and ensure a supply of vitamins A and C. Frozen juices stay indefinitely. Vitamin A can also be obtained in milk (this can be stored as powdered or evaporated milk if fresh milk tends to spoil before it is drunk), butter, margarine, and cheese. Cheese is also an excellent source of calcium, as are other dairy products.

3. Keep small cans of bean products on the shelves: chili, chickpeas, blackbean soup, and hot dogs and baked beans. These foods are good sources of folic acid, vitamin B_6, thiamin, riboflavin, potassium, and protein. They can be heated by putting the opened can in a pot of boiling water and then the contents eaten directly out of the can, thus minimizing clean-up. (A plastic spoon can be used to reduce further cleaning-up time.)

4. Other canned products (e.g., soups, ravioli, macaroni and cheese, tunafish, sardines, salmon, chicken, and meat spreads) are good foods to have for last-minute suppers or when you decide to eat at home but the supermarket is closed. Frozen foods are a source of a variety of nutrients. Frozen vegetables and fruits and fruit juices, frozen yogurt, frozen bran muffins, rice dishes, and complete dinners supply nutrients from one or more of the four food groups.

5. Nuts and seeds can be stored indefinitely and are fine sources of protein, zinc, iron (walnuts, sunflower and pumpkin seeds), and vitamin B_6.

6. When eating out, go to restaurants which serve vegetables and have salad bars. At the salad bar, fill up with dark green lettuce leaves, string beans, chickpeas, spinach, beets, green pepper, carrots, raw cabbage, and kidney beans. Order vegetables and baked potatoes rather than french fries (the baked potato has a higher vitamin C content than french fries).

7. Order milk when eating out, especially at fast-food restaurants or doughnut shops. This is important if the single eater avoids keeping milk at home.

8. Find friends who like to cook and who serve a variety of grains, vegetables, and dairy products. Eat with them as frequently as the friendship allows.

The Peripatetic Eater

It is difficult to meet one's nutritional requirements while traveling since one's food choices are often predetermined by the airline caterer or the availability of a highway food franchise. A regular traveler should consult his food record to see whether his traveling prevents him from obtaining his daily nutrient requirements. If so, he should consider the following suggestions to improve his diet.

1. Take advantage of the airline beverage service to obtain milk, orange juice, or tomato juice (or Bloody Mary mix) in addition to coffee, tea, and soda.

2. It is easy to obtain a variety of vegetables if one is traveling by air; simply order a vegetarian meal. These usually include yogurt, cheese, rice, occasionally a hardboiled egg, and of course a variety of vegetables. (They don't taste any worse than most economy class airplane meals.)

3. Breakfast is an excellent opportunity for the traveler to eat foods which may be missing from lunch and dinner. Motel, bus terminal, airport, and local daytime restaurants offer a variety of foods from several food groups. Citrus fruit juice, milk, hot cereal (e.g., oatmeal, cream of wheat), whole wheat toast, cold cereals, eggs, bran muffins, pancakes, and in certain geographic locations fresh fruit, bagels, hominy grits, and scrapple are usually available. Take advantage of this meal; you may be able to obtain several of your daily requirements and then

not have to worry if you are forced to eat lunch or supper at a stand-up counter at an airport or on the road.

4. If not inconvenient, carry small packages of seeds, nuts, raisins, or dried fruit so you have something nutritious to munch on if mealtime is irregular and the only foods available are candy bars and cookies.

Car travel expands the repertoire of the items that can be taken. In addition to the snacks already mentioned, fresh fruit, cheese (in cold weather), cold meat, sandwiches, and an insulated container of soup can be brought from home or replenished at a restaurant, thereby offering some alternative to eating at the ubiquitous fast-food franchises. (If food is put in an insulated bag that contains a frozen coolant, it is not susceptible to spoilage so long as the bag is cold. If you stay in a motel, you can refreeze the coolant in the ice machine.) Small cereal packages, cans of fruit (with pull-tab tops), and containers of tomato or orange juice can also be taken along to augment the menu selection at roadstand eating places.

Improving one's nutrient intake need not be difficult, inconvenient, or unpleasant. It simply takes knowledge about one's own eating habits, some advance planning, and motivation.

> An acquaintance who travels considerably and also must eat at work-related dinners and receptions has become adept at eating nutritionally well away from home. He always has a large breakfast: grapefruit, eggs, bran muffins or whole wheat toast, coffee, and milk. He skips lunch. He does this because the lunches available to him are usually sandwiches, hot dogs, hamburgers, or cold cuts, and he feels he does not need the calories and can get the other nutrients later in the day. If he gets hungry in the afternoon, he buys yogurt from a vending machine or lunch counter.
>
> At receptions and dinners, he heads toward the seafood bowl if available and fills up on shrimp on the theory that it is low in calories and high in minerals. He also eats all the carrot sticks, cherry tomatoes, and parsley that he can find (he is a caterer's nightmare as he consumes all the garnishes) and drinks a few glasses of tomato juice from the bar. He avoids anything with sauce, dips, spreads, or fillings, again to reduce his caloric intake. At the dinner itself, he asks the waitress for any extra salads (he assumes someone did not show up and the salad is sitting uneaten). He also asks for extras on vegetables (this is not always successful if the plates are filled in the kitchen). He avoids desserts unless he is eating in a restaurant (rather than a catered banquet) and can get fresh fruit. If he feels calcium-deprived because, for example, he did not have milk or yogurt during the day, he asks for a glass of milk.

The Athletic Eater

Adults who compete in athletic events on a regular basis, even as amateurs, may have special dietary needs. For example, food intake may be limited to easily digested foods so the stomach and upper intestine are empty during the competition. Food and water intake may be planned to prevent dehydration and feelings of hunger during the event. Some athletes drink liquid formulas that contain a meal's worth of protein, vitamins, minerals, and calories instead of eating solid food because they are easily digested and empty out of the stomach rapidly. The formulas were developed for patients who are unable to eat solid foods; Sustagen and Ensure are two examples.

Recently a system of eating to increase the amount of stored starch (glycogen) in muscle cells has become popular among participants in competitive events of intermediate length, e.g., a mile run, rowing contests, or wrestling matches (it is also followed by some marathon runners). The glycogen, normally stored in extremely small amounts in the muscle, can be converted to energy more quickly than fatty acids, the more commonly used energy source of muscle cells. According to anecdotes overheard at the Boston Marathon, its availability also decreases muscle pain. Increasing glycogen stores is done by first eating a low-carbohydrate diet for several days and then exercising vigorously; according to the theory, this uses up the glycogen in the muscles. A high-carbohydrate diet is then followed for a few days prior to the actual event (14).

Carbohydrate loading may have some benefits for the short-distance runner, but it is also associated with some definite risks. It may increase water retention in the muscle, which would result in a feeling of stiffness and heaviness. In the older athlete, cardiac pain and abnormalities in electrocardiograms have been found. This dietary regimen should be followed only with the advice of a physician.

For decades athletes have been eating excessive amounts of protein, vitamins, and minerals in the belief that these foodstuffs improve their performance. I once saw two downhill ski competitors take at breakfast pills from at least 2 dozen bottles of vitamin and mineral supplements. No scientific study has shown that these supplements have any effect on athletic performance, and indeed the excess consumption of nutrients stored by the body (e.g., the fat-soluble vitamins) can be harmful (15–17). Some athletes increase their protein consumption because of the mistaken belief that exercise "consumes" muscle and eating protein is the only way to replace it. Despite the absolute lack of evidence for this belief, large amounts of protein are still consumed. The recent availability of predigested liquid protein has started a new trend: Several ounces of this material are consumed a few hours before the competitive event with the expectation that, as an amateur wrestler said, "it will get into the muscles quickly and make them work better."

Food for Sport (18) is a useful book for those who want more information about dietary practices to be followed during training and competition. Additional references on the subject of diet and sport appear at the end of this chapter.

SPECIAL NUTRITIONAL NEEDS

The adult nutrient requirements listed in Table 1 may be insufficient for adult eaters who are pregnant, lactating, taking oral contraceptives, smoking or drinking heavily, or taking medications known to alter the availability of certain nutrients. Pregnant and lactating women need to increase their intake of many nutrients (19). Their needs are discussed in Chapters 5 and 6.

There is a great deal of controversy over whether women who take oral contraceptives need to increase their vitamin B_6 and folic acid intake. Women taking oral contraceptives should consult with their doctors about the adequacy of these vitamins in their diet; a list of recent reports on the subject is offered at the end of the chapter.

Cigarette smokers should be concerned about obtaining sufficient vitamin C in their diet. Studies have shown that eating about 45 mg[1] of ascorbic acid (the amount found in 4 ounces of orange juice, 10 strawberries, or one-half an orange) may not be enough for heavy smokers. A comparison of their serum vitamin C levels with those of the nonsmoker consuming the same amount of vitamin C showed the smokers to have much lower levels, even though their vitamin C intake was the same (20). Vitamin C intake for smokers should be about 100 mg (about 8 ounces) of orange juice, 20 strawberries, or a whole orange.

The need for increased nutrients because of medication should be checked with one's physician.

NUTRIENTS MOST OFTEN MISSING FROM THE DIET

Certain nutrients are consumed in inadequate amounts by the average American eater simply because the nutrients are found in foods which are often overlooked or eliminated from the diet. Three of the most common are calcium, folic acid, and iron. Calcium is easily obtained if one eats dairy products or dark green leafy vegetables such as kale, collard greens, beet greens, or mustard greens. Few of us include these vegetables in our daily diet, however.

There are two categories of dairy product consumers: those who drink a lot of milk and eat yogurt, cheese, cottage cheese, or even ice cream with some regularity; and those who never drink milk, dislike yogurt, think cottage cheese is only for dieters, and restrict their dairy food intake to cheese and an occasional ice cream cone.

> I have heard of people who turn to bones for their calcium supply. A colleague told me of a house guest who consumed entire chicken skeletons (cooked, of course). Her crunching on the bones became so irritating the host finally asked her to leave. He said: "We came into the kitchen to clean up after dinner and the plate which had contained the remains of the chicken was empty. She ate the bones like a beaver gnaws through wood; she really must have needed the calcium."

Those adults who eat neither dairy products, "greens," nor bones may be obtaining considerably less calcium than they need. A United States Department of Agriculture (USDA) survey of 5,500 women found that the calcium intake of women 45 and older was about one-half the required amount (21).

One consequence of chronic underconsumption of calcium may be osteoporosis. This disease is found among older women and is characterized by a decrease in the density of the bones and spontaneous fractures. Menopause and other related metabolic changes are probably also related to the development of

---

[1]This amount (45 mg) was the RDA for ascorbic acid in the 8th edition of the *RDA* (1974).

the disease. An insufficient intake of calcium along with the demands that pregnancy and nursing make on a woman's calcium stores contribute significantly to their depletion (21). (The disease is also found among men but less commonly.)

If it is extremely difficult to eat the calcium because of the incompatibility of one's eating style with those foods which contain it, then a calcium supplement should be considered. However, consult with a physician before starting one.

Folic acid intake can easily be inadequate if the daily diet consists of doughnuts for breakfast, hamburgers for lunch, and TV dinners for supper. Dark green leafy vegetables are an excellent source of folic acid, as are broccoli, asparagus, lima beans, kidneys, nuts, whole-grain cereals, and lentils. Good sources among foods the average eater might eat are folic acid-fortified breakfast cereal, wheat germ, and liver (it can be chopped). Relatively good sources include beer, cottage cheese, fresh peas and corn, and mushrooms. Although actual folic acid deficiency is rare today except among people with exceedingly restricted diets, it is certainly easy to eat slightly less than we need because some of the foods which contain folic acid are not routinely served in restaurants, are a bother to prepare, do not meet our tastes, or are expensive (asparagus and broccoli) unless one lives in an area where the foods are grown.

The best sources of iron are beef and liver. Since many Americans consume large amounts of these foods, iron deficiency should not be a problem. It is a problem, however, among people whose particular eating style eliminates these foods and some others that are iron-rich, such as other meats: lamb, pork, ham, chicken. Other nonanimal foods also contain iron: raisins, dried beans, seeds, nuts such as walnuts, and dark green leafy vegetables, but the iron in these foods is not as well absorbed as the iron in meat (eggs contain iron, but it also is not well absorbed). Some people avoid meat because of its fat content, to reduce caloric intake, its expense, or the time required to prepare it.

If your food intake record does not contain many iron-rich foods, one of the easiest ways of obtaining iron in absorbable form is to eat an iron-fortified cereal for breakfast or as a before-bed snack.

NUTRITIONAL CLAIMS, CONTROVERSIES, AND CONCERNS

Eating no longer seems to be a simple matter of making food choices compatible with our nutrient requirements and eating styles. It now seems important to select some foods because they contain some health-promoting quality and to avoid others because their consumption may lead to illness and even eventually to death. Thus it is not uncommon to find people eating large quantities of fiber, yogurt, brown rice, vitamin C, or molasses in the belief that any or all of these foods will make them "feel better" and to find the same individuals or others avoiding sugar, white bread, potato chips, soda, meat, and dairy products because they are afraid these foods will make them ill. Even those who have not committed themselves to an eating pattern influenced by these beliefs worry about whether they are causing themselves or their families harm by continuing to eat eggs, food with additives, or candy bars. This concern is exacerbated by the absence of clear and unambiguous recommendations from the scientific and medical communities, and the presence of confident assertions from self-appointed nutrition experts. Scientists are still working on the relationship between diet and heart disease, cancer, and high blood pressure. Either they make cautious and sometimes ambiguous nutritional recommendations, or they reverse recommendations made in the past. Meanwhile, nutrition "experts" are rushing into print with their confident assertions that garlic, ginseng, or yogurt cures all disease and brings about perfect health. Indeed it is extremely difficult to escape the proclamations of these "experts" since they appear on talk shows, and their statements are in books, magazines, and newspapers; furthermore, their views are communicated by friends and relatives at parties, on the bus, or in grocery stores.

> Nutritional advice has been given, unsolicited, since Adam and Eve.
> Then He asked, "Did you eat of the tree from which I had forbidden you to eat?" The man said, "The woman You put at my side—she gave me of the tree and I ate." And the Lord God said to the woman, "What is this you have done!" The woman replied, "The serpent duped me and I ate." Gen. 3:11–14 (22).

This section discusses some of the controversial areas in nutrition today and presents whatever conclusions are available from current scientific studies and government evaluations. Since information in this area is changing continually, the reader is cautioned to check the status of some of the conclusions drawn here against newly published scientific information. A list of books and periodicals that are current and reliable sources of nutritional information is provided at the end of the chapter for the reader who wishes to learn more in a certain area or check the resolution of a specific nutritional conflict.

During 1977 a controversial report was published by the now-defunct Senate Select Committee on Nutrition under the chairmanship of Senator George McGovern. The report, entitled "Dietary Goals for the United States" (23), set forth nutritional recommendations designed to improve the health of the American eater. The recommendations included:

1. Decreasing the number of calories from fat in the diet to 30% from the current intake of 40%, and eating only 10% of the fat calories in the form of saturated fats.

2. Increasing consumption of complex carbohydrates to 40 to 45% of daily caloric intake while reducing consumption of sugar (a simple carbohydrate) from 24 to 15%.

3. Keeping protein intake at 12% of the total caloric intake.

4. Reducing daily cholesterol intake to 300 mg (one egg contains 250 mg).

5. Reducing salt intake by 85% to about 3 grams a day.

The recommendations correspond rather closely with the type of diet we would obtain if we conscientiously ate all the grain, cereal, fruit, and vegetable servings recommended for the adult and were careful about the type of high-protein foods we consumed. The number of daily servings of meat, cheese, peanut butter, and eggs would have to be monitored very closely to avoid consuming too much fat or cholesterol. In addition, foods high in salt would be restricted, along with foods high in sugar.

Fat/Cholesterol

Foods which contain saturated fat include beef, cream cheese, nondairy creamers, whipped and light cream, cheese, ice cream, cottage cheese, yogurt (made from whole milk), eggs, butter, chicken fat, lard, herring, mackerel, eel, tunafish, salmon, carp, poultry, lamb, veal, nuts, pork, and solid vegetable shortenings and margarine made with hydrogenated oils.

Foods that contain over 100 mg of cholesterol (for 3 ounces) include tunafish canned in oil, lobster, shrimp, egg, liver, kidney, and brain (the latter contains 1,700 mg).

> The diet can be analyzed to estimate the amount of fat calories using the following method:
> 1. Keep a record of daily food intake. [*The Fat Counter Guide* (by R. Deutsch, Bull Publishing Co., Palo Alto, Calif., 1978) lists the percent of fat, carbohydrate, and total calories in most commonly eaten foods.]
> 2. Look up the fat content of each food in a food composition book. The information is listed as grams of fat per serving (or for 100 grams or 3 ounces of food).
> 3. Add up all the grams of fat eaten.
> 4. Multiply that number by 9; this converts grams to calories as each gram of fat contains 9 calories.
> 5. Divide the number of fat calories by the number of total calories eaten that day; multiply by 100. This number is the percent of daily calories represented by fat.

A revised edition of the McGovern report was issued in the winter of 1978 in answer to criticisms from the medical and nutritional community that the previous recommendations were inappropriately strict, might lead to nutritional deficiencies among certain age groups, were based on erroneous information, and had overlooked some obvious nutritional problems such as obesity and alcoholism.

The cholesterol levels were challenged by critics (24) who pointed out that the relationship between the diet and heart disease was only tenuously established, and many factors (e.g., smoking, high blood pressure, heredity, and, indirectly, obesity and exercise) may all be involved in the development of this disease. Although some studies have shown that a high intake of cholesterol results in an elevated concentration of cholesterol in the serum (25), several others have shown that this relationship may not hold when the levels of dietary cholesterol fall within the amounts normally eaten by the typical American (300 to 800 mg a day) (26–28). Moreover, eggs, which are the richest source of cholesterol in the diet, are also an excellent source of easily digestible protein and several vitamins and minerals. Recommending their elimination from the diet might lead to an inadequate nutrient intake among groups in the population whose diets are limited in animal protein, such as the elderly and young children (see Chapters 5, 6, and

7). Thus the new report eased the cholesterol restrictions for young children, the elderly, and premenopausal women (who are less susceptible to heart disease than men).

Salt

The rather strict recommendation to decrease salt intake found in the original report has also been eased; we are now told we may eat 5 grams (instead of 3 grams) each day. We normally consume 6 to 18 grams of salt a day, so even this larger permitted amount of salt may seem too little for some people.

Foods high in salt include bacon, bologna, corned beef, ham, luncheon meats, sausage, salt pork, salted herring, anchovies, sardines, peanut butter, canned boullion, catsup, spices with the word salt after them (e.g., celery salt), meat tenderizers, prepared mustard, relishes, processed cheese and spreads, strongly flavored cheeses (e.g., Roquefort), pickles, sauerkraut, potato chips, popcorn, pretzels, olives, and anything sprinkled with salt (e.g., salted bread sticks) (23).

Although we can consciously cut back on the amount of salt we add to our food, in order to be successful in reducing our salt intake, we must also be careful about eating highly salted foods and using salt or sodium-containing condiments and spices. Many people do not realize, for example, that celery, garlic, onion, and seasoning salts contain sodium, as does meat tenderizer and monosodium glutamate. (MSG is a flavor enhancer and is added to many prepared mixes. It is also sold as a cooking ingredient under the trade name Accent.)

The reason for decreasing salt consumption is to decrease the risk of developing hypertension, or high blood pressure. Although salt intake per se does not cause hypertension, it can elevate blood pressure in people who are genetically susceptible to this disease. People who have high blood pressure are usually told to stay on a low-salt diet. Hypertension is also found in some obese people, and a recent report (29) indicated that weight reduction was even more effective in reducing blood pressure than medication and a low-salt diet. (In fact, the people were encouraged to eat low-calorie salty foods like pickles to keep them on their diets.)

There is some debate over whether a decrease in salt consumption is beneficial to those without a tendency toward high blood pressure; some physicians and scientists feel that salt intake is unimportant in the development of this disease in people whose blood pressure is unaffected by salt consumption.

However, it may be difficult or even impossible for the average American to reduce his intake of salt to even 5 grams a day. Since there is no medical evidence that exceeding this amount causes high blood pressure in people who are not genetically predisposed (30), an eater who has just finished a bowl of salted peanuts or a dill pickle does not have to run and check his blood pressure. However, reducing salt consumption certainly is not dangerous or harmful and may, if one has inherited the tendency to have high blood pressure, be beneficial.

Sugar

The McGovern Committee recommended a reduction in the intake of refined sugar. In the original report the Committee recommended dropping sugar consumption to 15% of total caloric intake. The revised edition drops it further, to about 10% of total caloric consumption. We now eat about 24% of our total caloric intake in the form of refined sugar. Eating sugar has clearly been related to the development of dental caries (31). Therefore it makes economic as well as nutritional sense to eat less sugar.

There is, however, nothing inherently dangerous about sugar despite the claims of some people who write books saying that it causes psychiatric problems (32). [For a comprehensive review of all scientific studies on the relationship between the sugar and disease, see the report done for the FDA (31). this report states that sugar does not *cause* heart attacks, cancer, schizophrenia, or criminal behavior. It does cause bacteria to grow on the teeth, and this results in cavities.] Sugar also contributes calories to our diet because it is found in a large category of pleasurable foods—desserts and snacks. These foods taste good, especially to those who have a "sweet tooth," and are often consumed simply for the pleasure of eating them. Unfortunately they often give more than pleasure: They are likely to contribute extra calories to our diets and eventually extra pounds. Decreasing our sugar intake thus theoretically may help control weight, although the causes of overeating are usually more complex than our passion for chocolate chips or hot fudge sundaes (see Chapter 8).

Many foods that contain sugar contain few other nutrients. (Sugar is a nutrient; it is a carbohydrate and contributes energy to the diet.) This lack would not be a nutritional problem if these foods were regarded as extras in our diet rather than staples. Desserts, which usually contain sugar, are not thought of as the major nutritional contribution of a meal (although some people still think it is the only part worth eating), and no one would expect to meet his nutrient needs by eating dessert. However, when sugar-rich, nutrient-poor foods are eaten as the main component of a meal or snack (doughnuts for breakfast, a candy bar for lunch, an ice cream sandwich in the middle of the afternoon) the eater is depriving himself of foods which do supply needed nutrients. The presence of the sugar itself does not contribute to the nutrient-poor diet; the consumption of sugar-rich foods instead of foods from the four food groups does.

> Recently, as I was waiting for a trolley during the evening rush hour, my ear caught the sound of crunching. Being hungry, I turned to see who was eating and found myself staring at a fellow passenger who was eating some peanut brittle. During the subsequent 10-minute wait, he ate another piece of peanut brittle, a chocolate bar, and two pieces of chocolate marshmallow fudge. My thoughts ranged from offering him nutritional resuscitation with a carrot to wondering whether he would eat dinner after his three-course candy snack.

Sugar is a natural constituent of many foods: milk, fruit, certain vegetables, honey, maple syrup, sorghum, sugar cane, molasses, and sugar beets. Sucrose, the sugar we usually eat directly as table sugar, is made up of two sugar molecules: fructose and glucose. Fructose is the sugar found in fruits, and glucose in a slightly modified form (dextrose) comes from corn and is found, for example, in corn syrup. Lactose is the sugar present in milk, both human and cow.

Sucrose comes from either sugar cane or sugar beet. White sugar is sucrose that has been refined to remove impurities and color. Brown sugar is sucrose that still contains molasses. The molasses syrup–sugar mixture is boiled until only sugar crystals are left and is then centrifuged. Brown sugar is also produced by adding molasses to white sugar. Brown sugar is the same in taste and nutritional quality regardless of how it is processed.

Raw sugar is the sucrose obtained after the sugar cane juice is evaporated. It is only 96% pure (white sugar is 99% pure) and contains soil, fibers, molds, yeasts, bacteria, lint, and waxes.[2]

Honey is formed by an enzyme (honey invertase) from nectar. The source of nectar (clover, orange blossoms) affects the color and taste of honey. Honey contains the following sugars: 38% fructose, 31% glucose, 1% sucrose, and 9% a mixture of other sugars. It also contains 17% water and minimal amounts of thiamin, riboflavin, and ascorbic acid (vitamin C). Honey and brown sugar contain calcium, phosphorus, and iron, but brown sugar contains slightly more. Neither is a practical source of nutrients other than energy.

Molasses is a thick liquid which is formed during the processing of sugar cane or beets. It comes in different grades. The highest is *edible molasses,* which contain sugar, iron, and a few other nutrients found in brown sugar. *Blackstrap molasses* is the final extract of molasses and contains the same nutrients found in edible molasses.

Corn syrup is made from the starch in corn. It contains dextrose (the commercial name for glucose), fructose, maltose, and some other sugars. Corn syrup is used primarily in food processing.

Although some of the sugar we consume is in the form of table sugar added to beverages, cereals, or fruit or as an ingredient in foods baked at home, we eat almost as much as an additive in processed foods. Sucrose and other sugars are used in food processing as a sweetener, but they also have several functions unrelated to taste. Some of these are listed in Table 7. The taste of processed food is not a reliable indicator of its sugar content. Some breakfast cereals such as the bran family (Bran Flakes, All Bran, Bran Buds, 100% Bran) contain more sugar than Sugar Frosted Flakes (All Bran contains 20%; Frosted Flakes, 15.6%) (33). Yet if one were to judge the sugar content of the cereal by its sweetness, most people would assume Frosted Flakes contained the greater amount. Although most food labels do not list the content of sugar by weight or as a percent of the total ingredients, its position in the list of ingredients on the label provides some idea of its relative concentration in the food. If sugar is among the first two or three ingredients listed, it can be considered to be a major component of the food; if it comes toward the end, it probably is present in small amounts, and the food should not be considered a "sugar-rich" food.

---

[2]There is a purified "raw" sugar product now available: Kleenraw. It is made from 97% sucrose to which molasses is added; the mixture is then crystallized to form the large crystals characteristic of raw sugar.

TABLE 7. *Common uses of sugar*

1.	Sweetener.
2.	Increases the growth of yeast in baked goods (housewives add sugar to yeast and water to "proof it").
3.	Delays coagulation of protein. Used in recipes which require heating eggs without coagulating or curdling them (custards, souffles, egg cream sauces).
4.	Sets jams and jellies by combining with the pectin in fruit.
5.	Prevents molds from forming in jams and jellies owing to its high concentration.
6.	Prevents the formation of large ice crystals in frozen foods. Maintains the firmness of frozen foods.
7.	Necessary for the fermentation of beer and homemade wines.
8.	Provides bulk and texture to a variety of foods such as beverages, cakes, and ice cream.
9.	Sugar syrups maintain the flavor and texture of canned foods.

The relative concentration of sugar in the following product is obvious—it is listed as the first ingredient.

"10-Second Tomato Soup" (distributed by Nestlé Company, Inc.). Ingredients: sugar, tomato powder, food starch-modified, salt, hydrogenated vegetable oil, natural flavors, dehydrated onion, lactose, garlic powder, artificial flavor, sodium caseinate, monosodium glutamate, dipotassium phosphate, soy flour, mono- and diglycerides, artificial color, chicken fat, chicken meat, thiamin hydrochloride, sodium silicoaluminate, disodium inosinate, disodium guanylate, tricalcium phosphate lecithin, turmeric, corn syrup solids, spices, polysorbate 60.

Foods do not have to be avoided simply because they contain sugar; often it is present in such small amounts its caloric contribution is insignificant. For example, a package of Herb-Ox instant broth and seasoning, beef flavored, lists sugar as the third ingredient after hydrolyzed vegetable protein and salt. Seven ingredients follow. According to its place on the label, one might assume that the sugar and hence caloric content of the broth was high; however, an 8-ounce serving contains only 8 calories, and some of those calories come from the vegetable protein. (Protein and sugar each provide 4 calories per gram.) However, if sugar is the major ingredient of a food which is being eaten as a source of nutrients, not as dessert, unless the food has some other redeeming nutritional value it should be replaced with something more nutritious.

It is common to hear people claim that eating sugar causes a variety of unpleasant symptoms such as inability to concentrate, fatigue, dizziness, and faintness. These people claim to have "low blood sugar," a condition called hypoglycemia. Hypoglycemia is not uncommon. A health survey done with several hundred normal young adults indicated that about 25% of them had responded to a glucose tolerance test with low blood sugar (34). A glucose tolerance test is one in which the person drinks a concentrated solution of glucose and has the blood levels of glucose and insulin measured at frequent time intervals thereafter. Moreover, hypoglycemia has been found to be associated with an enormous variety of diseases, including disorders of the liver, nervous system, intestinal tract, and endocrine glands; cancer; and severe exercise in a starved and alcholic person; it also occurs after insulin administration in diabetes (34). The hypoglycemia seen in these cases, however, is usually associated with other physical symptoms and not primarily with the cluster of unpleasant psychological sensations referred to earlier.

Studies of people with simple hypoglycemia indicate that: (a) it may be the prelude to diabetes; (b) it is not related to food habits or the specific consumption of carbohydrate foods; (c) the unpleasant symptoms associated with it are absent in many people who show a low blood sugar with the glucose tolerance test; and (d) many of those who have the psychological symptoms did not experience them at the time their glucose tolerance test indicated their blood sugar level was low (34).

It has been suggested that some of the symptoms ascribed to hypoglycemia may be related to stress or anxiety, and diet alone may not be sufficient to correct them. Although a low-carbohydrate diet has been advocated as treatment, physicians have been cautioned not to substitute a high-protein diet for a carbohydrate one since eating protein enhances insulin secretion and it is insulin which lowers blood sugar (34). Often a combination of diet therapy and psychological support are necessary to relieve the symptoms.

Fiber

If the adult eater consciously reduces his consumption of highly processed foods and instead eats a variety of grains (rice, buckwheat groats, bulgur), beans (kidney, chickpeas, black-eyed peas, lima beans), vegetables, and fruits, he will be eating more fiber. The dietary goals of the Senate Select Committee emphasize the importance of fiber in the diet, and indeed this nondigestible portion of plant food is receiving considerable attention as a necessary part of our food intake.

Interest in fiber was stimulated several years ago by the observations of epidemiologists that tribesmen in Africa have a lower incidence of certain diseases than their kinsmen living under more-modern urban conditions. The major difference between the two groups was their fiber intake (35). The rural population, who consumed about 50 grams of fiber a day largely in the form of vegetable products, seemed to have little or no appendicitis or diseases of the colon (diverticulosis, polyps, cancer), and a smaller incidence of heart disease, diabetes, and hiatus hernia (35). Further research indicated that it was difficult to tell whether the fiber itself was responsible for the absence or low incidence of these diseases or if other characteristics of a high-fiber diet were responsible, such as a lower consumption of animal protein, saturated fat, and calories; a higher consumption of complex carbohydrates (starch); production of bulkier, faster-moving stools; or even increased chewing time (36).

There is general agreement that a high-fiber diet helps relieve constipation and some problems associated with difficult or infrequent bowel movements (hiatus hernia, varicose veins, hemorrhoids). Diverticulosis, another intestinal tract disorder, has been helped in some people by increased fiber consumption (37).

The relationship of high-fiber intake to other diseases such as cancer of the colon or heart disease must be studied further since some additional epidemiological information has confused the situation. For example, appendicitis, once thought to be associated with a low-fiber diet, has been steadily declining in this country and Britain. Moreover, women in these two countries complain of constipation (a sign of a low-fiber diet) more than men; yet colonic cancer is found as frequently among men as women. Finns, who consume very little dietary fiber but large amounts of dairy products, have a low incidence of colonic cancer and a high incidence of heart disease. Despite the absence of compelling evidence that eating fiber-rich foods makes us live longer, it is agreed on by the medical community that a high-fiber diet does relieve constipation and increases our consumption of vitamins and minerals since these nutrients are commonly found in high-fiber foods.

A reasonable fiber intake is 30 to 60 grams a day (36). Good sources of fiber include: bran, carrots, cabbage, nuts, celery, blackberries, dried apricots, raisins, figs, artichokes, popcorn, green pepper, peas, peanuts, sesame seeds, winter squash, broccoli, prunes, raspberries, rice, buckwheat groats (kasha), bulgur, dried beans, and sunflower seeds.

It is not necessary to calculate the number of grams of fiber in the diet. If these high-fiber foods are substituted for highly refined foods in the diet, changes in bowel movements and the size of the stool will indicate the presence of sufficient fiber.

One word of caution for those who are switching from a low-fiber to a high-fiber diet: It can decrease the amount of certain minerals which are absorbed from the intestinal tract into the bloodstream because dietary fiber contains substances (e.g., phytates) that bind or hold onto these minerals. In extreme cases this binding or interference with the absorption of these minerals can lead to deficiencies. The minerals affected by the high-fiber diet are calcium, magnesium, and zinc. If the following foods are included in the diet, these minerals should be well supplied: dairy products and dark green leafy vegetables for calcium: dried beans, nuts, peanuts, wheat germ, coffee, cocoa, and chocolate for magnesium; and meat, nuts, wheat germ, and shellfish for zinc.

VITAMIN AND MINERAL SUPPLEMENTS: THEIR PLACE IN THE AMERICAN DIET

People have been taking vitamin and mineral supplements for years; most of the supplements contain nutrients in amounts equivalent to the RDAs. They are taken from habit, as nutritional insurance against an inadequate supply of nutrients from the diet, to prevent coming down with a cold or the flu, to shorten the duration of respiratory illness, and often when the eater is overworked, tired, stressed, or on a diet.

Taking vitamins and minerals in this quantity is not harmful and can be beneficial for the casual eater who cannot remember at the end of the day whether he drank orange juice for breakfast or had any dark green leafy vegetables for supper. They compensate for some nutritional deficiencies in the diet and are useful for the busy, peripatetic, single or negligent eater. It would be better nutritionally for such an eater to follow the suggestions at the beginning of the chapter and alter his eating pattern so the needed nutrients can be eaten in the diet rather than swallowed in a pill.

Many people, however, take vitamin and mineral supplements who do not require them. Before starting or continuing on vitamin and mineral pills, the individual should spend a week or so monitoring his food intake as outlined earlier to determine if he is actually deficient in any nutrient.

Vitamin and mineral supplements are not a substitute for a good diet. They do not contain many of the trace minerals the body requires; they certainly do not contain any of the nutrients whose requirements are just now being estimated; and they do not contain fiber, essential fatty acids, and protein. Food still remains the best source of nutrients.

There have always been a group of people who believe that extremely large quantities of vitamins and minerals must be consumed in order to stay healthy. Recently their numbers have been growing in conjunction with the number of health food stores, which supply them with these nutrients. [An excellent and very readable discussion on this is found in *The New Nuts Among the Berries* (38).] The nutrients are consumed in megadoses, about 10 times or more the required amounts. Vitamin C is probably the most widely consumed vitamin in mega-quantities. Linus Pauling and others have been advocating the consumption of large amounts of vitamin C as a way of preventing colds and flu for several years. For almost every known nutrient, there is someone who advocates its consumption in megaquantities. This advice is usually given in periodicals and paperbacks written for people who are concerned with food and health. Frequently this information is given out in newspaper columns, talk shows, and newsstand magazines.

> The only way to feel the full impact of this trend toward consuming large amounts of nutrients is to go to a health food store. Look at the labels on the bottles of supplements, read some of the brochures promoting them, and talk to the salespeople and customers. (The salesperson in a health food store has replaced the corner druggist as the dispenser of "over-the-counter" medical advice.) The reasons people give for buying particular nutrients vary, but most are related to the belief that the consumption of a nutrient or combination of nutrients will make the person feel better or will prevent him from coming down with a cold, diabetes, cancer, arthritis, or heart disease. Ironically, many people who buy such supplements eat nutritionally excellent diets. Some people believe, however, that by the time the food is harvested, processed, packaged, and prepared, it loses most of its nutrients and thus cannot be relied on as a source of nutrients. They may also believe that their particular nutrient needs are far in excess of the amounts that can be supplied easily by food.

Evidence for the efficacy of meganutrients can be found in the countless testimonials from people who were cured by these nutrient supplements and in warnings by the authors of books and articles about the diseases we shall suffer if we do not take them.

Many of the ailments that should be treated with nutrients are those which many people experience at some time: insomnia, burping, "blue Mondays," constipation, poor posture, fatigue, forgetfulness, bloodshot eyes, and chapped lips. An individual is often made to feel as if he is suffering from a variety of nutritional deficiencies when he reads books like *Let's Eat Right To Keep Fit* by Adelle Davis (39). The symptoms associated with deficiencies in various nutrients are listed, and these ailments are so common that after reading the book many people are impelled to go to a health food store and buy some vitamin or mineral supplements. (Who among the readers has not felt tired, irritable, or stiff, or had chapped lips?) Although Davis extols the virtue of eating wholesome food, she says that food itself is unable to provide nutrients in the quantities needed for a healthy body. Hence one needs nutritional supplements. Once started, these supplements are apt to become a permanent part of the diet. Often the symptoms which stimulated their ingestion in the first place disappear (we stop feeling tired, or the chapped lips go away) when the supplements are taken. Although this can be coincidence, it is tempting to believe that their disappearance is due to the supplements. Often people continue to take the supplements because they believe their symptoms will return if they stop. If the symptoms return anyway (we are often tired, and in the winter often get chapped lips) the response is usually to take even larger amounts. The individual who is taking these supplements may start to read the monthly health-oriented periodicals which report on current nutritional research and its role in health. He may learn about his "need" for additional nutrients through these magazines or find out that due to his consumption of supplement X his body now requires supplemental amounts of nutrient Y. Thus he often finds himself taking several types of nutritional supplements each day.

Are these nutrients effective in preventing or curing disease? Are they dangerous? It is difficult to answer the first question definitively since much of the support for the use of large amounts of nutrients as medicine comes from personal anecdotes. If someone says he felt "like a new person" after taking large amounts of a particular vitamin, for example, or that his muscle ache, skin rash, arthritis, or insomnia went away, he should be believed. The symptom or problem probably did go away. However, there is only one way to know whether it was the nutrient or something else such as a placebo effect which made him feel better. (A placebo effect is the effect of believing that a therapy will help or that a doctor or faith healer has the power to cure.) This influence is extremely strong, and most physicians know scores of people who were "cured" of an ailment even when there was no effective therapy. (A dermatologist told me of a man who cured himself of warts after all known treatments had failed. He told himself the warts would go away and they did !) The only way to test the effectiveness of a nutrient (or any other medicine) for treating a medical problem is to do a double-blind study. In such a study neither the patient, doctor, or other staff member knows who is receiving the medicine and who is receiving the look-alike "sugar pill." Usually the patients are given the experimental treatment for several weeks or months and then are switched to the placebo (without their knowledge). The other group, who were receiving the placebo, are switched at the same time to the medicine. If the therapy works, its effectiveness should stop when the patients are no longer receiving it and are getting the placebo instead, and it should start helping the group who had been receiving the placebo.

Many diseases go away spontaneously. Often belief in the curative powers of an untested therapeutic agent (a vitamin, mineral, chicken soup) is reinforced by these unexplained, unexpected cures.

Double-blind experimentation has been done to test the effectiveness of vitamin C in reducing the frequency and severity of colds. A study with Navajo schoolchildren showed that no difference in the frequency or duration of colds and respiratory illness existed among those who were getting 1 gram of vitamin C (ascorbic acid) a day and those who were getting a placebo (40). Another study with adults found the same noneffect (41), and a third study (42) carried out with identical twins found a slight reduction in the severity of some of the cold symptoms among the young girls in the group but no other beneficial effect. Moreover, giving 2 grams of ascorbic acid to adult volunteers each day reduced the bacteria-killing activity of their white blood cells, which might prolong a bacterial illness (43).

Zinc has received attention lately, as several reports indicated that it may reduce some of the lesions of acne (44,45). (There is some preliminary evidence that acne may involve deficiencies of zinc and vitamin A.) Large doses of zinc also have been shown to reduce some of the symptoms of rheumatoid arthritis (46) and sickle cell anemia (47,48). This work is still very new, and it is important to remember that the amounts of zinc used in these studies are far greater than the nutrient requirements. Researchers are using the mineral as a drug, and it should not be taken in these large amounts without medical supervision (49).

Vitamin A has been shown to be effective in preventing the development of certain skin or epithelial cancers (skin, respiratory tract, mammary gland, bladder) in laboratory animals. Eventually this work might lead to ways of preventing similar types of cancer in humans. One problem in using vitamin A for this purpose now is that the doses are so great they would be harmful to us. Current research is focusing on developing and using synthetic vitamin A-like compounds that do not have the toxicity of vitamin A when given in large doses. Unfortunately, no one knows at this time whether these vitamin A-like compounds are helpful in the treatment of established cancers (49).

All of these nutrients are administered in extremely large quantities to determine their usefulness in treating disease. Although there is no conclusive evidence that any other nutrient is useful as a drug, it is always possible that other diseases will respond to large amounts of certain vitamins, minerals, or even amino acids.

This brings us to the second question: Are megadoses of these nutrients dangerous? The answer is: They can be (50). Like any drug, these nutrients, when ingested in megadoses, can produce side effects; and like any drug, in some people these side effects can be unpleasant, dangerous, and even life-threatening. For example, there is now evidence that megadoses of vitamin C can precipitate gout in people who have a tendency toward this disease, and can cause a type of anemia in some American Blacks, Sephardic Jews, Orientals, and other ethnic groups who carry a genetic defect affecting a particular serum (blood) enzyme (glucose-6-phosphate dehydrogenase). If a pregnant woman takes megadoses of vitamin C, her newborn child can develop scurvy. Any adult who has been taking megadoses of vitamin C is also susceptible to something called "rebound scurvey" if he decreases his intake of the vitamin to normal amounts (50).

The average adult suffers 1.1 colds a year. The studies on vitamin C show that this figure can be reduced only by about 36% at best if a person takes megadoses of the vitamin continually (51). Considering the hazards of the side effects, a person might weigh the benefits (having 0.84 colds a year) against the risks.

Side effects are also known to accompany excessive consumption of vitamin E: headaches, nausea, fatigue, dizziness, blurred vision, inflammation of the mouth, and gastrointestinal disturbances (51); and vitamin A: fatigue, bone or joint pain, abdominal discomfort, night sweats, loss of body hair, brittle nails, dry scaly rough skin, mouth fissures, and swelling of the arms and legs (and sometimes death). Vitamin D and calcium in excessive amounts can cause elevated serum levels of calcium, which can lead to kidney damage (51); in infants excessive vitamin D intake leads to loss of appetite, nausea, weight loss, and failure to thrive (51). Excessive amounts of folic acid can lead to seizures among susceptible individuals (49). There are also known side effects for megadoses of iron, zinc, and vitamin B_6.

If vitamins and minerals are taken in quantities considerably in excess of nutrient requirements, they pass out of the category of nutrients and into the category of drugs. They should be taken with the same caution and medical supervision as any drug. They should *not* be self-prescribed any more than an antibiotic or any other medication would be.

> If you encounter a physician who practices something called *orthomolecular (or holistic) medicine,* you should realize that his therapy may consist primarily of giving megadoses of vitamins and minerals. Although there is always the possibility that your condition may respond to this therapy, it is a good idea to seek another medical opinion, since this type of therapy is considered by most of the medical profession to be experimental and unproved.

There is no biological difference between natural vitamins and those synthesized in the laboratory. Both are used in identical ways by the body. Do not pay more for a vitamin because the label says "natural"; the only "natural" way to get a vitamin or mineral is to eat the foods which contain them (and for vitamin D, to expose one's skin to the sun).

EVALUATING EMERGING NUTRITIONAL CLAIMS AND CONTROVERSIES

This chapter and Chapter 7 cover most of the current controversies in nutrition. The information presented, however, has limited utility since it deals only with the information available at the time of its writing. The reader is still left to handle the continuous barrage of *new* nutritional claims and controversies that fill the newspapers, magazines, and airwaves. These claims demand the eater's attention. They suggest that his eating should change or that he at least worry about changing it. How do we know what to believe and if we should react? How do we discriminate between the sense and nonsense of nutritional theories and controversies? The following suggestions may help the eater to discriminate between nutritional fact and fiction.

1. Try to read regularly some of the periodicals and newsletters which report new developments in nutritional research and to review the status of controversial nutritional theories (such as the relationship between diet and heart disease). Some of these publications also discuss government regulations related to the use of food additives, food labeling, marketing and advertising, and nutritional intervention programs.

Most of these publications are available in public libraries or can be obtained from university or government libraries through interlibrary loan. Some are free and can be obtained by writing to the agency or foundation which publishes them. Others are inexpensive to subscribe to and might be worth getting on a monthly basis. All of these are listed at the end of the chapter.

2. Newspaper columns are sometimes a valuable source of basic and controversial nutritional information. The syndicated column by Jean Mayer and Johanna Dwyer is an example of a well-researched, carefully documented presentation; others, unfortunately, may be less accurate or try to promote a particular point of view. (The column written by Carleton Fredrick is an example of this.)

3. Obtain information, if possible, about the background and training of those who write articles for the popular press. Look for the following credentials.

(a) Does the writer have training and work experience in the fields of nutrition, medicine, dietetics, public health?

(b) Is he a spokesman for industry, government, or consumer advocate groups? This does *not* disqualify anyone from being taken seriously; however, by knowing the background of the author, the reader can evaluate the statements for possible, even unconscious, bias and then seek out statements by a spokesman representing another point of view. For example, a statement can be made by someone representing industry saying that certain foods are not acceptable unless they are artificially colored (margarine, for example). A consumer advocate group, who wants all additives removed from food, may state that the American eater should learn to eat natural (white) margarine. A third statement may come from a regulatory agency claiming that there is no known harm in eating yellow margarine, but perhaps the consumer should be given the choice of eating colored or uncolored margarine. You, the eater, can then weigh these statements and decide which are applicable to your own eating style and beliefs.

(c) Has the author or spokesperson published articles that are reviewed and evaluated for their scientific accuracy? If he has published articles in scientific journals, they will have been scrutinized by others in the same field. If he has published only in a newsletter put out by an agency (of which he may be the head) or if he has only written books, there is no guarantee that what he has written has ever been evaluated for its scientific credibility. You can obtain this information by writing to the author or to his publishing house or agency and asking for his bibliography.

(d) Are there references that support the author's statements? Sometimes these cannot be provided (as in newspaper columns) owing to lack of space. However, reputable columnists are always willing to provide a list of the original scientific articles from which they took their information.

(e) If the source of information is verbal (i.e., you are told some new nutritional "fact" by a co-worker, taxi driver, proprietor of a local store, or your sister-in-law), where did the communicator of such information hear about it? If the source was a television talk show or some other casual source, check it out further before accepting it. If there is nothing to read on the subject, call the dietetic department of your local hospital, the nutrition or home economics department of your local college, the food editor of your newspaper, or the consumer division of the FDA (there is a branch in most large cities); or go to the library and ask the librarian to help you find some material on the subject. The information may be correct; however, if it is going to make a radical change in your eating habits, it is worth spending some time making sure it is valid. You probably would not accept casual information about modifying the way you maintain or drive your car without checking it out with a reliable car mechanic. Since you cannot trade in your body, it is certainly wise to spend as much time checking the accuracy of information on how to maintain it so it "runs a long time."

Eating should not be a source of anxiety, worry, or guilt (unless you just ate three helpings of chocolate cake!). It is hard to eat wrong if a small amount of attention is paid to the nutritional quality of food choices. There is no perfect diet; man evolved in such a way that he is able to survive on widely varying diets; the "perfect" diet for a Fiji Islander would not be similar to the "perfect" diet of an Afghanistani. There is an immense variety of foods that can satisfy our nutrient needs. For the American eater, there is also a large variety of foods which satisfy every need except the nutritional one. The key to successful eating is to eat abundantly from the first group and very moderately from the second. An occasional candy bar, hot fudge sundae, blueberry pie, or potato chip will not bring about your nutritional downfall. Just eat prudently of these foods and watch out for serpents bearing apples.

REFERENCES

1. Food and Nutrition Board (1979): *Recommended Dietary Allowances,* 9th ed. National Academy of Sciences, Washington, D.C. *(in press).*
2. Sauberlich, H. (1973): Pantothenic acid. In: *Modern Nutrition in Health and Disease,* edited by R. Goodhart and M. Shils. Lea & Febiger, Philadelphia.
3. Goodhart, R. (1973): Biotin. In: *Modern Nutrition in Health and Disease,* edited by R. Goodhart and M. Shils. Lea & Febiger, Philadelphia.
4. Li,T-K., and Vallee, B. (1973): The biochemical role of trace elements. In: *Modern Nutrition in Health and Disease,* edited by R. Goodhart and M. Shils. Lea & Febiger, Philadelphia.
5. Hambridge, K. M. (1974): Chromium nutrition in man. *Am. J. Clin. Nutr.,* 27:505.
6. Mertz, W. (1975): Effects and metabolism of glucose tolerance factor. *Nutr. Rev.,* 33:129.
7. Li, T-K. (1973): Manganese. In: *Modern Nutrition in Health and Disease,* edited by R. Goodhart and M. Shils. Lea & Febiger, Philadelphia.
8. Nielson, F. H., and Sandstead, H. H. (1974): Are nickel, vanadium, silicon, fluorine, and tin essential for man? A Review. *Am. J. Clin. Nutr.,* 27:515.
9. Li, T-K. (1973): Molybdenum. In: *Modern Nutrition in Health and Disease,* edited by R. Goodhart and M. Shils. Lea & Febiger, Philadelphia.
10. Lappé, F. M. (1971): *Diet for a Small Planet.* Ballantine Books, New York.
11. Kushi, M. (1977): *The Book of Macrobiotics: The Universal Way of Health and Happiness.* Japan Publications, Elmsford, N.Y.
12. *Nutritional Analysis of Food Served at McDonald's Restaurants.* Warf Institute, Madison, Wis., 1977.
13. Kahn, P. (1976): One and two-member household feeding patterns. *Food Product Technol.,* 10:28.
14. Editorial Staff (1975): Nutrition and athletic performance. *Dairy Council Dig.,* 46:7.
15. Consolazio, C. F. (1971): Nutrition and athletic performance. In: *Progress in Human Nutrition,* edited by S. Margen. Avi Publ., Westport, Conn.
16. Astrand, P-O. (1967): Diet and athletic performance. *Fed. Proc.,* 26:1772.
17. Nelson, R.A., and Gastineau, C.F. (1974): Nutrition for athletes. In: *The Medical Aspects of Sports,* edited by T. T. Craig. AMA, Chicago.
18. Smith, N. (1976): *Food for Sport.* Bull Pub. Co., Palo Alto, CA.
19. Committee on Maternal Nutrition, Food and Nutrition Board (1970): *Maternal Nutrition and the Course of Pregnancy.* National Academy of Sciences, Washington, D.C.
20. Yeung, D. (1976): Relationships between cigarette smoking, oral contraceptives, and plasma vitamins A, E, C, and plasma triglycerides and cholesterol. *Am.J. Clin. Nutr.,* 29:1216.
21. Albanese, A. (1977): Osteoporosis. In: *Contemporary Nutrition,* Vol. 2, edited by A. Sloan. Nutrition Dept., General Mills, Minneapolis.
22. The five books of Moses, In: *The Torah.* The Jewish Publication Society, Philadelphia, 1962.
23. Select Committee on Nutrition and Human Needs, *Dietary Goals for the United States.* Government Printing Office, Washington, D.C., 1977.
24. Harper, A. (1977): Perspective: U.S. dietary goals. *J. Nutr. Educ.,* 9:152.
25. Shorey, R., Brewton, L., Sewell, R.D., and O'Brien, M. (1974): Alteration of lipids in a group of free living adult males. *Am. J. Clin. Nutr.,* 27:268.
26. Kannel, W.B., and Gordon, T. (1970): *The Framingham Diet Study: Diet and Serum Cholesterol.* DHEW, Washington, D.C.
27. Nichols, A.B., Ravenscroft, C., and Lamphiear, D.E. (1975): Daily nutritional intake and serum lipid levels: The Tecumseh study. *Am. J. Clin. Nutr.,* 29:1384.
28. Porter, M., Yamanaka, W., Carlson, S., and Flynn, M. (1977): Effect of dietary egg on serum cholesterol and triglyceride of human males. *Am. J. Clin. Nutr.,* 30:490.

29. Reisin, E., Abel, R., Modan, M., Silverberg, D., Eliahou, H., and Modan, B. (1978): Effect of weight loss without salt restriction on the reduction of blood pressure in overweight hypertensive patients, *N. Engl. J. Med.*, 298:1.
30. Food and Nutrition Board (1979): *Recommended Dietary Allowances, 9th ed.* National Academy of Sciences, Washington, D.C. *(in press)*.
31. Life Sciences Research Office (1976): *Evaluation of the Health Aspects of Sucrose as a Food Ingredient.* Fed. of American Societies for Experimental Biology, Bethesda.
32. Rodale, J.I. (1968): *Natural Health, Sugar, and the Criminal Mind.* Pyramid, New York.
33. Shannon, I. (1974): Sucrose and glucose in dry cereals. *J. Dent. Child.*, 12:17.
34. Danowski, T.S., Nolan, S., and Stepahn, T. (1975): Hypoglycemia, *World Rev. Nutr. Diet.*, 22:288.
35. Burkitt, D.P., Walker, A.R.P., and Painter, N.S. (1974): Dietary fiber and disease. *JAMA*, 229:1068.
36. Mendeloff, A. (1977): Dietary fiber and human health. *N. Engl. J. Med.*, 297:811.
37. Bing, F. (1976): Dietary fiber in historical perspective. *J. Am. Diet. Assoc.*, 69:498.
38. Deutsch, R. (1977): *The New Nuts Among the Berries.* Bull Publishing Co., Palo Alto, CA.
39. Davis, A. (1970): *Let's Eat Right to Keep Fit.* New American Library, New York.
40. Coulehan, J., Eberhard, S., Kapner, L., Taylor, J., Rogers, K., and Gary, P. (1976): Vitamin C and acute illness in Navajo schoolchildren. *N. Engl. J. Med.*, 295:973.
41. Elwood, P.C., Lee, H.P., St. Leger, A.S., Baird, I., and Howard, A.N. (1976): A randomized trial of vitamin C in the prevention and amelioration of the common cold. *Br. J. Prev. Soc. Med.*, 30:109.
42. Miller, J., Nance, W., Norton, J., Wolen, R. Griffith, R., and Rose, R. (1977): Therapeutic effect of vitamin C: A co-twin study. *JAMA*, 37:248.
43. Sheotri, P., and Bhat, K. (1977): Effect of megadoses of vitamin C on bactericidal activity of leukocytes. *Am. J. Clin. Nutr.*, 30:1077.
44. Michaelsson, G., Juhlin, L., and Vahlquist, A. (1977): Effects of oral zinc and vitamin A in acne. *Dermatology*, 113:31.
45. Michaelsson, G., Vahlquist, A., and Juhlin, L. (1977): Serum zinc and retinol-binding protein in acne. *Br. J. Dermatol.*, 96:283.
46. Simkin, P.A. (1976): Oral zinc sulphate in rheumatoid arthritis, *Lancet*, 2:539.
47. Prasad, A.S., Ortega, J., Brewer, G.J., Oberleas, D., and Schoomaker, E.B. (1976): Trace elements in sickle cell disease. *JAMA*, 235:2396.
48. Anonymous (1977): Sickle cells shape up with zinc. *Med. World News*, 18:42.
49. Weininger, J., and Briggs, G. (1977): Nutrition update. *J. Nutr. Educ.* 9:173.
50. Herbert, V. (1975): The rationale of massive dose vitamin therapy. In: *Proc. West. Hemisphere Nutr. Congress IV*, p. 84, Sciences Group, Acton, Mass.
51. Herbert, V. (1977): Megavitamin therapy. In: *Contemporary Nutrition*, Vol. 2, edited by A.E. Sloan. Nutrition Dept., General Mills, Minneapolis.
52. Smith, E. (1975): A guide to good eating the vegetarian way. *J. Nutr. Educ.*, 7:109.

RECOMMENDED READING

General

1. *Recommended Dietary Allowances,* National Academy of Sciences, 9th edition, 1979.
   Available from the Printing and Publishing Office, National Academy of Sciences, 2101 Constitution Ave., Washington, D.C. 20418 *(in press)*.
   This inexpensive book contains readable summaries of the nutrient needs of different age groups and the requirements during pregnancy and lactation. It contains current references on nutrient requirements and the most recent information on nutrients whose requirements have not yet been completely determined.
2. *Dietary Goals for the United States,* Select Committee on Nutrition and Human Needs, United States Senate, February 1977.

Available from the Superintendent of Documents, Government Printing Office, Washington, D.C. 20402. Stock No. 052--3913-2, Catalog No. Y4.N95:D63/3.

A good source of information on the fat, cholesterol, and salt content of common foods. Also contains a comprehensive discussion on the current American diet, its relation to health, and recommendations for changing dietary intake.

3. *FDA Consumer,* Food and Drug Administration. Published monthly except July-August and December-January when one issue is released. It is found in most public libraries.

Subscription rate $10/year. Write to U.S. Superintendent of Documents, Washington, D.C. 20402.

This magazine contains articles of general interest on the safety of foods, drugs, and cosmetics: explains current government regulations in these areas; discusses subjects of nutritional controversy; and explains the function of the FDA. The back of the magazine lists seizures of foods, drugs, and cosmetics that fail to meet safety and labeling standards.

4. *Nutrition Today,* edited by C. Enloe, Nutrition Today, Inc., 101 Ridgely Ave., Annapolis, MD. 21404.

Free monthly magazine available after joining Nutrition Today Society. Membership open to concerned laymen. Subscription rate $14.00/year. May be available in some public libraries and university libraries.

Excellent source of current information on nutritional research and controversies. Also contains well-written articles on history of food and nutrition, and explanations of the function of nutrients in the body.

5. *Federal Register,* Office of the Federal Register, National Archives and Records Service, General Services Administration, Washington, D.C. 20402

This bulletin is available in government agency libraries and should be available in most large public libraries. Subscription rate $50/year.

This publishes the regulations and legal notices issued by federal agencies. Good source of information on legislative action related to government-supported nutrition intervention programs.

6. *Parents' Magazine,* Parents' Institute, Bergenfield, N.J. 07621.

Subscription rate $9.95/year. Available in most public libraries and newstands.

This magazine contains articles on health and nutrition; the articles are written by well-recognized experts and are a reliable source of information and advice. Occasionally articles of general interest appear, although most of the topics are concerned with pregnancy and child-rearing.

7. *CNI Weekly Report,* Community Nutrition Institute, 1146 19th St. N.W., Washington, D.C. 20036.

Subsciption rate $25/year. At present available only by direct mailing.

This is a weekly publication which reports on all legislative activity on food and nutrition. Unlike the *Federal Register,* the activities are reported in understandable language rather than legal terminology; pending legislation and activities by government agencies are also reported. Occasionally the editorial comment is biased against industry, the scientific community, or government. However, the reporting is accurate and up-to-date.

8. *The Wall Street Journal,* Dow Jones and Co., New York, N.Y. 10007.

Subscription rate $49/year. Available from The Wall Street Journal, Dow Jones and Co., Chicopee, Mass. 01021. Also available on the newstands and in most large public libraries.

This newspaper regularly reports on nutritional issues and research.

9. *Dairy Council Digest,* National Dairy Council, Rosemont, Ill. 60018.

Free newsletter, available to educators and health professionals, and probably to concerned laymen. Call local Dairy Council office to be on mailing list or write to national headquarters at 6300 N. River Rd., Rosemont, Ill. 60018.

Well-written and referenced articles on matters of nutritional concern. Articles are *not* restricted to subjects of concern to the Dairy Council and are totally unbiased.

10. *Contemporary Nutrition,* edited by A.E. Sloan, General Mills, Minneapolis.

Free newsletter. Available by writing to Nutrition Dept., General Mills, Inc., P.O. Box 1113, Minneapolis, Minn. 55440.

Similar to *Dairy Council Digest* in scope and accuracy of articles.

11. *Journal of Nutrition Education,* 2140 Shattuck St., Suite 1110, Berkeley, CA. 94704.

Available in many university libraries and through inter-library loan. Subscription rate $12/year.

This contains mainly articles on nutrition education; however, all current nutritional concerns of interest to the general public are usually discussed throughout the year, including a valuable "nutrition update" article. Inexpensive and free, written and audiovisual materials are listed each month, and several reviews of publications appropriate for different audiences are included.

12. *Food Values of Portions Commonly Used,* C. Church and H. Church, 12th ed., Lippincott, Philadelphia, 1975.
13. *Nutritive Value of Foods,* USDA Home and Garden Bulletin, No. 72, 1977, Government Printing Office, Washington, D.C. 20402.
    References 12 and 13 are excellent sources of information on the caloric and nutrient composition of foods. They include information on multi-ingredient foods (e.g., sandwiches, stews) as well as single-ingredient foods.
14. *The Harvard Medical School Health Letter,* Dept. of Continuing Education, Harvard Medical School, 25 Shattuck St., Boston, Mass. 02115.
    Issued monthly. Subscription rate $12/year.
    This newsletter contains accurate and current information on matters of general health; however, articles are frequently included on nutritional issues such as the use of megavitamins, fiber, or diet and heart disease.
15. *The New Nuts Among the Berries,* R. Deutsch, Bull Publ. Co., Palo Alto, CA. 1977.
16. *Health Foods, Facts, and Fakes,* S. Margolius, Walker and Co., New York. 1973.
    References 15 and 16 are excellent sources of information on current fashions in eating, food faddism, and nutritional quackery.
17. *The Consumer's Right to Know,* Kraft, Inc., Dept. D, 500 N. Peshtigo Ct., Chicago, Ill. 60690.
    Single copies free.
    Pamphlets and booklets on subjects ranging from recent government legislation on food additives and labeling to basic nutritional information; they are easily understood, attractively packaged booklets. Excellent source of material for personal use, classroom teaching, or work with community groups.
18. *Consumer Reports,* Consumers Union of the United States, Inc., Mt. Vernon, New York.
    Issued monthly. Subscription rate $11/year.
    Analyses of the nutrient content of commonly eaten foods (fast foods, processed foods) appear occasionally and provide useful and practical information.

Oral Contraceptives and Nutrient Intake

1. Horwitt, M., Harvey, C., and Dahm, C. (1975): Relationship between levels of blood vitamins C, A and E, serum copper compounds, and urinary excretions of tryptophan metabolites in women taking oral contraceptive therapy. *Am. J. Clin. Nutr.,* 28:403.
2. Larsson-Cohn, U. (1975): Oral contraceptives and vitamins. *Am. J. Obstet. Gynecol.,* 121:84.
3. Leklem, J.E., Brown, R., Rose, D., and Linkswiler, H. (1975): Vitamin B_6 requirements of women using oral contraceptives. *Am. J. Clin. Nutr.,* 28:535.
4. Leklem, J., Linkswiler, H., Brown, R., Rose, D., and Anand, C. (1977): Metabolism of methionine in oral contraceptive users and control women receiving controlled intakes of vitamin B_6. *Am. J. Clin. Nutr.,* 30:1122.
5. Lindenbaum, J., Whitehead, N., and Reyner, G. (1975): Oral contraceptive hormones, folate metabolism and the cervical epithelium. *Am. J. Clin. Nutr.,* 28:346.
6. Margen, S., and King, J. (1975): Effect of oral contraceptive agents on the metabolism of some trace minerals. *Am. J. Clin. Nutr.,* 28:392.
7. Miller, L., Johnson, A., Benson, E., and Woodring, M. (1975): Effect of oral contraceptives and pyridoxine on the metabolism of vitamin B_6 and on plasma tryptophan and amino nitrogen. *Am. J. Clin. Nutr.,* 28:846.
8. Miller, L.T., Dow, M.J., and Kikkeler, S.C. (1978): Methionine metabolism and vitamin B_6 status in women using oral contraceptives. *Am. J. Clin. Nutr.,* 31:619.
9. Newman, L.J., Lopez, R., Cole, H.S., Boria, M.C., and Cooperman, J.M. (1978): Riboflavin deficiency in women taking oral contraceptives. *Am. J. Clin. Nutr.,* 31:247.
10. Nordquest, M., and Medved, E. (1975): A nutrition counseling session for college women on the pill. *J. Nutr. Educ.,* 7:29.
11. Pietarinen, G., Leichter, J., and Pratt, R. (1977): Dietary folate intake and concentration of folate in serum and erythrocytes in women using oral contraceptives. *Am. J. Clin. Nutr.,* 30:375.

12. Prasad, A., Oberleas, D., Lei, K., Moghussi, K., and Stryker, K. (1977): Effect of oral contraceptive agents on nutrients. I. Minerals. *Am. J. Clin. Nutr.,* 30:377.
13. Smith, J., Goldsmith, G., and Lawrence, J. (1975): Effects of oral contraceptive steroids on vitamin and lipid levels in serum. *Am. J. Clin. Nutr.,* 28:371.

Vegetarian Eaters

1. Brown, P.T., and Bergan, J.G. (1975): The dietary status of 'new vegetarians.' *J. Am. Diet. Assoc.,* 67:455.
2. Dept. of Nutrition, School of Health, Loma Linda University, Loma Linda, CA 92354. They have many publications on vegetarian diets.
3. Erhard, D. (1971): Nutrition education for the 'now' generation. *J. Nutr. Educ.,* 3:135.
4. Goldbeck, N. (1972): *Cooking What Comes Naturally.* Cornerstone Library, New York.
5. Goldbeck, N. and Goldbeck, D. (1975): *The Dieter's Companion.* New American Library, New York.
6. Guley, H. (1977): A vegetarian program for students on a college board plan. *J. Am. Diet. Assoc.,* 69:236.
7. Lappe, F.M. (1971): *Diet for a Small Planet.* Ballantine Books, New York.
8. Raper, N., and Hill, M. (1973): *Vegetarian Diets,* Nutrition Program News, U.S. Dept. of Agriculture, July-August.
9. Robertson, L., Flinders, C., and Godfrey, B. (1976): *Laurels Kitchen.* Nilgiri Press, Berkeley.
10. Smith, E. (1975): A guide to good eating the vegetarian way. *J. Nutr. Educ.* 7:109.

Macrobiotic Eaters

1. *Food Composition Table for Use in East Asia* (1972): National Institute of Arthritis, Metabolism, and Digestive Diseases, NIH, Bethesda, Md. 20014.
2. Kushi, M. (1977): *The Book of Macrobiotics: The Universal Way of Health and Happiness,* Japan Publications, Elmsford, New York. This book can be obtained in stores which sell food and other items to the macrobiotic community.
3. *Selected Bibliography on East Asian Food and Nutrition* (1972): National Institute of Arthritis, Metabolism and Digestive Diseases, NIH, Bethesda, Md. 20014.
4. The macrobiotic community has study houses in which a novice can learn about the macrobiotic diet.

Nutrition for Athletes

1. Bergstrom, J., and Huetrnan, E. (1972): Nutrition for maximal sports performance. *JAMA,* 221:991.
2. Committee on Nutritional Misinformation (1974): Water deprivation and performance of athletes. *Nutr. Rev.,* 32:313.
3. National Dairy Council (1974): Nutrition and athletic performance. *Dairy Council Dig.* 46:7.
4. Slovic, P. (1975): What helps the long distance runner run? *Nutr. Today,* 10:18.
5. Smith, N.J. (1976): *Food for Sport,* Bull Publishing Co., Palo Alto, CA.

APPENDIX

Pantothenic Acid

The vitamin pantothenic acid is found in a wide variety of foods. The best sources include meat, chicken, cereals, peanuts, pecans, walnuts, cauliflower, avocados, sweet potatoes, eggs, dates, and prunes. Most vegetables, fruits, dried beans, dairy products, fish, and enriched flour contain this vitamin so a pantothenic acid deficiency is very rare.

The vitamin forms part of a multipurpose enzyme complex, coenzyme A, and takes part in reactions involving, for example, the formation of acetylcholine (a nervous system chemical messenger); the synthesis of fatty acids, cholesterol, sterols (substances which form the reproductive hormones); and in reactions resulting in the production of energy-containing compounds (2).

Biotin

Biotin is a vitamin that is found in most natural foods; the best sources include egg yolks, liver, tomatoes, and yeast. Raw egg white contains a substance, avidin, which combines with biotin and prevents its absorption from the intestine. However, a biotin deficiency is unlikely to occur unless large quantities of raw egg white are consumed (3).

Biotin is involved in enzymatic reactions which transfer carbon dioxide among substances in the cell (carboxylation reactions). For example, it transfers carbon dioxide (CO_2) to a compound (malonyl-CoA) involved in the synthesis of fatty acids; it also transfers CO_2 in a series of reactions that result in the formation of energy-containing compounds (ATP).

Vitamin K

Vitamin K is discussed in the chapter on the nutritional needs of the infant.

Copper

Copper is a mineral that forms part of an important system of enzymes which comprise the final steps of the formation of the high-energy compound ATP. It is a constituent of a pigmented enzyme called cytochrome oxidase (4). Copper is important in hemoglobin formation and seems to promote absorption of iron from the intestinal tract. It is also involved in the transport of iron into the bloodstream. (It participates in changing (oxidizing) iron so it is picked up by a special protein that carries it through the bloodstream.) It is essential for the normal development of the central nervous system and connective tissue, e.g., cartilage. Moreover, it is part of other enzyme systems, including one responsible for the pigmentation of the skin (4). Copper is widely distributed in foods; the best sources are: nuts, oysters, clams, liver, raisins, and dried beans.

Chromium

Chromium is found in most grains, molasses, and Brewer's yeast. The refining of sugar, milling of wheat, or cooking of vegetables in a lot of water (which is then thrown away) substantially reduces chromium content. Beer, black pepper, liver, beef, and mushrooms are also good sources of chromium.

This mineral exists in the body as a complex with nicotinic acid (a compound formed from the vitamin niacin) and certain amino acids. This complex is called the glucose tolerance factor (GTF). GTF works with insulin, a hormone responsible for regulating blood levels of glucose. It is thought that GTF might promote the action of insulin by binding it to cell membranes inside and outside the cell (5).

A chromium deficiency produces symptoms similar to those seen with insulin deficiency in diabetes, and chromium has been given to diabetics to improve their ability to handle glucose. Chromium levels are very low among some middle-aged and elderly individuals in this country; although the significance of this is still unclear, it may be a factor in the development of diabetes seen among elderly individuals (6). Chromium has been given to some elderly people with impaired glucose tolerance and in some cases has improved their condition.

Chromium supplementation is most effective when GTF is used rather than the mineral itself. Not all foods that contain chromium contain GTF. For example, egg yolks contain high concentrations of chromium but not GTF (6).

Manganese

Cereals, soybeans, legumes, nuts, tea, and coffee are the best sources of manganese. This mineral apparently is poorly absorbed by the small intestine; in this particular way it is like iron, and therefore its content in foods may not be related to the amount actually entering the body. Its absorption is inhibited by high levels of calcium and phosphorus (accompanying, for example, a high intake of dairy foods).

Manganese is part of many enzyme systems (4), including those involved in the formation and breaking down of certain amino acids, in the incorporation of certain types of sugar molecules (xylose and galactose) into a carbohydrate–protein compound which forms part of cellular membranes, in maintaining the structural properties of ribonucleic acids (cellular compounds involved in protein synthesis), and in the formation of urea (the compound used to remove excess nitrogen from the body)(7).

Fluorine

Fluorine was discovered during the late 1930s to have a beneficial effect on the prevention of dental caries. Thirty years later it was also found to decrease the incidence of bone disease such as osteoporosis and others in which bone demineralization (loss of minerals) occurs (8).

The most reliable dietary source of this mineral is fluoridated water; seafoods and tea are also high in fluorine, and cereal and other grains contain smaller amounts (8).

Molybdenum

Molybdenum, a mineral, is found as part of many enzyme complexes, some of which also contain iron (9). Among the reactions in which it is involved are those in which hydrogen is transferred from a donor to a recipient molecule (oxidation–reduction). One such enzyme, xanthine oxidase, functions in the liver to remove hydrogen (a process called oxidation) from a number of nitrogen-containing substances so they can be processed for excretion from the body.

Molybdenum is found in legumes (dried beans), whole grains, milk, and leafy vegetables.

Selenium

Selenium, another mineral, is a constituent of the enzyme glutathione peroxidase, which prevents the breakdown of fatty acids into undesirable compounds. Like vitamin E, selenium thus helps stablize membranes containing fatty acids against compounds known as oxidants. The mineral is taken up from the soil by plants and is found in whole grain and cereal products (4).

3 *THE EATER AS CONSUMER*

Primitive man had great difficulty obtaining safe and nutritious food. He could be killed by the animal he was hunting; he might be poisoned by the food he was gathering; and he had no way of knowing whether the foods he ate met his nutrient needs. Although the only immediate physical danger confronting today's consumer while gathering his food is being hit by a shopping cart, he faces the problem of selecting foods that satisfy his nutrient needs, and he worries about the safety of the foods he eats. Unfortunately, the modern supermarket offers few guidelines to help him make nutritious and safe food choices.

Most supermarkets are overwhelming. The shopper, dragging his weary feet up and down the aisles, tries his best to select wisely from among more than 12,000 items, but he may come to believe that only a committee from the Food and Drug Administration (FDA) could make nutritionally and economically astute food purchases.

The modern shopper can get by without being an expert on food processing, labeling, and nutrition; but it is a frustrating fact of life that nutritionally wise food shopping requires time, effort, and a lot of patience. Few of us have these virtues to draw on while food shopping. Some people read the newspaper the evening before shopping and note the weekly food specials; others free themselves from making any decisions by buying many of the same items week after week. As a result we: (a) tend to ignore many nutritionally valuable items; (b) fail to compare the nutrient content of a highly processed item with the nutrients in the same item prepared from scratch; and (c) trustingly assume that a particular product's ingredients never change.

> A woman never noticed the whole-wheat flour sitting on the shelf in the baking goods section until she attended an adult education course in nutrition. She learned there about the considerable nutritional difference between white and whole wheat flours, and now she uses the latter for cake, pancake, muffin, and cookie batters.
>
> Another woman thought that dried peas and beans were useful only for her children's art projects (they glued the beans to cardboard to make "mosaics"). When they outgrew this pastime, she fed these vegetables to the local squirrels. Her interest in dried beans and peas reawakened when her son became a vegetarian and told her about their high protein content. The next time she went to the supermarket, she noticed an entire shelf filled with bags and boxes of dried legumes. In over 20 years of shopping at this supermarket, she had never before stopped to examine them.
>
> A third shopper bought a variety of prepared foods every week or two and never bothered to read the ingredients listed on the label. One day her daughter investigated the labels for a school nutrition project. She pointed out to her mother that sugar was the major ingredient in the cereal, salt in the dried soup, sugar in the hot chocolate mix, and water in the cheese spread. She went with her mother to the supermarket and

showed her that certain ready-to-eat cereals did not contain sugar as the major ingredient and that canned soups did not have a lot of salt. She also suggested adding chocolate syrup to milk instead of using a dried cocoa mix as the latter contains considerably less calcium, more sugar, and no vitamin A or D. Finally, at home she showed her mother how to make a water-free cheese spread by beating cheese in a blender. The mother, impressed but still uncommitted to label reading, pleaded bifocal fatigue and asked her daughter to take care of reading all the food labels in the future.

Food should be bought with care; since the shopper is the one bringing food into the family, he should feel a special responsibility for making nutritionally sound purchases. Doing this requires an investment of time to obtain information about the products we usually buy and to become familiar with products we usually overlook. This knowledge cannot be acquired at 5:00 p.m. when supper has to be on the table at 6 p.m., or the day before Thanksgiving, or when a blizzard is coming and everyone is nervously stocking up on milk and candles. I recommend spending an extra half-hour or so every 3 or 4 months to investigate the supermarket. Labels can be read and compared, unfamiliar foods looked at and considered for purchase, and processed foods (frozen and dried) carefully judged for their nutritional value as well as their convenience.

This chapter provides the background necessary for understanding nutritional labels, interpreting ingredient labels, and evaluating the utility of food additives. Some of the recent controversies over certain additives in food are also discussed.

NUTRITIONAL LABELING

Foods often have a nutritional label and an ingredients label. A nutritional label is legally required if: (a) the product is enriched or fortified with vitamins, minerals, or protein; (b) a nutritional claim is made for the product either by advertising or on the package itself (e.g., if the product is said to be important for growth and health); or (c) the fat content or calories are listed (then the rest of the nutrient information must be provided).

Some manufacturers add nutritional labels to their products voluntarily. Of course, suppliers of fresh meat and produce find nutritional labeling difficult or impossible (it would necessitate analyzing each individual cabbage, pork chop, or flounder for size, water content, fat content, and so on).

Table 1 shows the nutritional label found on a package of breakfast cereal. The information can be interpreted as follows:

1. *Serving size and number of servings per container:* The serving size is a rough guess at how much of the food an average male who engages in light activity is likely to eat. It is assumed that the particular food will be eaten as part of a meal (rather than the entire meal). All the nutritional information is given in terms of one serving size.

2. *Calories:* This information enables the shopper to select foods that have a high nutrient-to-calorie ratio. For example, he might find that one serving of a fruit-flavored juice contains the same calories as one serving of canned grapefruit juice, but the grapefruit juice has many more nutrients; or that a fruit-flavored yogurt contains many more calories than plain yogurt but does not contain any

TABLE 1. *Nutritional label from a box of Cheerios (General Mills)—1978*

Nutrition Information Per Serving	
Serving size	1 ounce (1¼ cups)
Servings per container	10

	1 oz Cheerios	Cheerios plus ½ cup vitamin D milk
Calories	110	190
Protein (grams)	4	8
Carbohydrate (grams)	20	26
Fat (grams)	2	6
Percentage of U.S. Recommended Daily Allowances (U.S. RDA)		
Protein	6	15
Vitamin A	25	30
Vitamin C	25	25
Thiamin	25	30
Riboflavin	25	35
Niacin	25	25
Calcium	4	20
Iron	25	25
Vitamin D	10	25
Vitamin B_6	25	30
Vitamin B_{12}	25	35
Phosphorus	15	25
Magnesium	10	15
Zinc	6	8
Copper	8	8

more nutrients. Some shoppers base their selections on calorie content alone: the lower, the better. This method is not wise because it leads to the exclusion of many nutritionally valuable foods and the selection of other foods which contain primarily water. The question is: "Am I getting my calories' worth of nutrients if I buy this product?"

3. *Nutrient content:* After the calories, the label shows the amounts (in grams) of protein, carbohydrate, and fat found in one serving. The label then lists other nutrients (and protein a second time) as a percent of the U.S. Recommended Daily Allowance (U.S. RDA).[1] For example, one serving of Cheerios without

---

[1]The U.S. RDA is a simplified version of the RDA. The RDA lists the nutrient requirements for (both sexes) infants, children, and adults, and for pregnant and lactating women. The U.S. RDA uses the nutrient requirements for adult men listed in the RDA (as they are the highest of any category) to establish standards for the nutrient content of foods, except that iron requirements are based on female needs as they are higher than for males.

There are actually four U.S. RDAs: one for adults, one for infants under 12 months of age (this appears on baby foods), another for use on "junior" foods, and another for foods formulated for pregnant and nursing women.

The U.S. RDA for proteins is slightly complicated because of the difference between vegetable and animal proteins. Animal proteins (found in meat, milk, and eggs, for example) amply provide the essential amino acids—substances the body needs and cannot adequately make on its own. Plant proteins are low in certain essential amino acids and are also less digestible than animal protein. We must therefore eat relatively large quantities of plant protein in order to obtain the essential amino acids we require. Thus 10 grams of milk protein supplies 22% of the U.S. RDA, whereas 10 grams of plant protein (e.g., the protein in rice or cornflakes) supplies only 15% of the U.S. RDA. The U.S. RDA for animal protein is 45 grams, for plant protein 65 grams.

milk (Table 1) supplies about 4 grams of protein. According to the U.S. RDA, we need 65 grams of vegetable protein per day; one serving of Cheerios, without milk, therefore supplies about 6% of the U.S. RDA (4 grams = 6% of 65 grams). Other nutrients listed are vitamins A and C, thiamin, riboflavin, niacin, calcium, and iron. This information is required on all nutritional labels; the manufacturer has the option of including vitamins D, E, B_6, and B_{12}, folacin (folic acid), biotin, pantothenic acid, phosphorus, iodine, magnesium, zinc, and copper.[1]

The label also includes the carbohydrate and fat content of the food. Sodium and cholesterol contents may be listed as well; although no regulation makes mandatory provision of the latter information, this may change shortly. Some manufacturers voluntarily put the sugar content on labels so the shopper can see how much of the carbohydrate is made up of sugar.

The nutritional label shows how well a food meets our daily nutrient needs and which nutrients the food lacks. It is particularly useful in evaluating highly processed foods; for example, if a hypothetical can of spaghetti with tomato and meat sauce contains texturized food starch, imitation tomato flavor, and soy rather than beef protein, its nutrient content is lower than that of another can containing tomato sauce made from tomatoes and meat made from meat. The shopper can see the difference by reading the nutritional label—he need not try to translate the list of ingredients on the label into nutrient values.

Foods are fortified with vitamins and minerals for different reasons. In some cases (such as the addition of vitamin D to milk or B vitamins to breads and pasta) the addition substantially improves our nutrition. On the other hand, the enrichment of snack foods (especially sweet ones) is what cynics call "the nutritional horsepower race" since it is done to give the products a competitive edge. A shopper is more likely to select a cupcake for his child that is vitamin-C fortified than one that is not. Shoppers should take a second look at the nutritional labels on these products; in many cases the label reveals that the amounts of added nutrients are small (usually in the range of 2% to 10% of the U.S. RDA), and if a shopper really wants to add nutrients to the family diet he should forget about the cupcakes and head for the produce or frozen orange juice. These products that have the same or more nutrients for fewer calories.

Some products are fortified with a large variety and quantity of nutrients. These foods (primarily diet foods and the breakfast cereals, drinks, and bars) have been classified as dietary supplements by the FDA as they contain between 50% and 150% of the U.S. RDA for several nutrients. These products have more nutritional value than the sparsely fortified snack foods; indeed the nutrient supplementation is similar to that provided by a vitamin–mineral pill.

The shopper should nevertheless keep two things in mind regarding the nutritional value of added nutrients. The first is that even fortified snack foods rarely substitute for fruits, vegetables, grains, dairy products, meat, fish, or eggs in nutritional value. The second is that foods fortified with a vitamin pill's worth of nutrients are worthwhile only when the shopper cannot obtain these nutrients elsewhere. Fortified foods do not contain the trace nutrients (substances that are necessary in small amounts) found in a variety of grains, beans, vegetables, fruits, and proteins; and often they lack fiber. (Bran cereal, for example, contains fewer nutrients than some other cold cereals, but it is an excellent source of fiber.) Heavily fortified foods should therefore not be eaten just to give the eater license to consume nutritionally empty food for the rest of the day.

INGREDIENT LABELING

The only way to obtain information about some foods is by reading their ingredient labels. The following information should be kept in mind.

1. Do not be dismayed if some foods do not have an ingredient label. There is a category of foods that follow a standard recipe in their preparation. The ingredients, which are agreed on by the FDA and the food manufacturers, are listed in the *Federal Register,* a government document that reports FDA regulations and is available in federal and some public libraries. Since it is not convenient to go to the library before shopping, it is fortunate that many manufacturers of these products voluntarily put the ingredients on their labels.

2. Ingredients are listed in the order of their concentration. The following ingredients appear on a package of instant onion-flavored broth: hydrolyzed vegetable protein, onion, salt, sugar, vegetable fat, tomato, celery, caramel, garlic, disodium inosinate, disodium guanylate. The vegetable protein is present in the highest concentration; the rest are present in progressively smaller amounts according to their order on the label.

The name of a food product also indicates the relative concentration of its ingredients and can be very revealing. If the name on the package is "meatballs and gravy," it contains more meatballs than gravy. If the name is "gravy and meatballs," the consumer should realize that gravy makes up the larger portion.

It is important for people who must restrict their salt or sugar intake to be aware that ingredients are listed in the order of their concentration. Such people should be especially careful to read labels since salt and sugar appear in suprising places and amounts. For example, a random reading of the labels of some popular dehydrated single-portion soup mixes revealed many which listed salt as the *first* ingredient, and others that listed sugar first.

3. Highly processed foods are being manufactured today with imitation ingredients to reduce their cost. Unless the consumer reads the label, he cannot know that traditionally used ingredients were replaced by imitation ones.

A recent report in *Food Products Development* (2), a trade magazine for food processors, described new products designed to replace cocoa powder and thus offer "significant savings to food processors." These products contain modified food starch, soy flour, soybean oil, palm oil, cottonseed oil, artificial and natural flavorings, and artificial coloring. Next to the description is a picture of a plate piled high with chocolate cupcakes, cream-filled chocolate bars, and chocolate-covered, marshmallow-filled cookies. A consumer would have no reason to suspect that these familiar items are not what they used to be unless he reads the label.

The label on a box of frozen pepperoni pizza lists the following ingredients under "tomato sauce": dehydrated tomato flakes, modified starch, potato flour, mono-sodium glutamate, sugar, beet powder, citric acid, artificial certified color. The pizza shown on the cover of the box has melted cheese surrounding pepperoni circles, but the "cheese," according to the label, actually consists of "imitation mozzarella cheese (water, saturated soya oil, potassium caseinate, salt, lactic acid, lipolyzed butter oil, potassium sorbate, artificial certified color)" and a small amount of actual mozzarella cheese (3).

Aside from changing the taste and texture of foods, imitation ingredients alter the nutrient content. The substitution of food starch for tomatoes, and soy flour and palm oil for mozzarella cheese, in a pizza decreases its nutritional value. (Real tomatoes contribute vitamins A and C and potassium; cheese contributes calcium, riboflavin, and protein; modified food starch and soybean flour contribute primarily calories.)

Not all convenience foods use imitation ingredients. The consumer should determine which products still contain ingredients with good nutritional value, so he obtains some nutrients along with convenience. (A suggestion: bring gloves or mittens to the supermarket to wipe frost from the frozen food packages; otherwise cold hands may curtail your label reading in this department.)

4. Canned foods now contain information unavailable a year ago. The weight of the drained solids (that is, the solid food with the packing liquid removed) is now listed. This information is very useful since the difference between the weights of drained and undrained food may be 3 to 4 ounces.

5. Recently the National Canners Association decided to use "open code dating" on canned goods. This means that cans now have a date that indicates when the food was processed or when it should be sold or consumed. Breakfast cereals have had this notation for years, as have dairy products; but until recently the only way the consumer could know when a canned food was still edible was to break the code in which the date was written. This information will be most useful to the homemaker deciding whether to use a long-forgotten canned food unearthed after shelf cleaning or unpacking after a move. The notation may be a date that corresponds to the date of packaging, or the date may be accompanied by such words as "use by" or "sell by."

6. The FDA requires food manufacturers to identify the type of fat or oil used in a product. Food labels must now state whether the fat comes from beef or lard, for example, or whether the oil is soybean, coconut, or safflower. In addition, the oils must be described as saturated, partially saturated, or unsaturated. This information is especially useful to consumers who want to reduce their consumption of saturated fats and oils.

SHOPPING TIPS

1. Shop the periphery of the supermarket first. Purchase the meats, fish, produce, dairy products, frozen foods, and baked goods before doing other shopping. Then enter the inner aisles, selecting those which contain canned

goods, cereals, baking goods, spices, grains, dried beans, pet foods, powdered milks, ethnic foods, and cleaning and paper goods. If possible, avert your eyes while walking past crackers, soda, candy, cookies, and boxes of highly processed entrees and desserts.

2. Before going through any aisle, ask yourself if any of the foods there are really necessary. A pause at the head of the aisle featuring soft drinks, potato chips, or fruit-flavored powder may be sufficient to eliminate that aisle entirely.

3. Do not shop when hungry or when accompanied by anyone who is hungry.

4. Before buying a highly processed convenience food, read the label and decide whether the benefit of the convenience is high enough to compensate for any nutritional loss.

5. Make regular attempts to buy a nutritious food that you have been passing by because you were prejudiced against it, someone in the family claimed to dislike it, or it was unfamiliar. Liver, yogurt, wheat germ, lima beans, kale, fresh fish, bran cereal, brown rice, and sardines are a few examples of foods that might be overlooked or discounted. Try these and other foods from the four food groups at least once; someone might like them, and they might even become staples.

6. Look at the food items in the shopping carts of your fellow shoppers. Do this while standing in the checkout line because there is time then to ask your fellow shopper about items with which you are unfamiliar or to get suggestions on how to cook a particular product. (People love to give advice!)

NUTRIENT LOSSES

Food processing exacts its toll on nutrients. As a general rule, the more steps a food goes through between harvest and consumption, the greater are its nutrient losses. Many nutrients are removed as a potato is transformed into a potato chip, wheat into macaroni twists, or corn into cornflakes. One of the most striking examples of nutrient loss occurs as whole wheat flour goes through the additional step which transforms it into white flour. The following nutrients are lost: 70% of vitamin B_6, 50% of pantothenic acid, 66% of folic acid, 86% of vitamin E, 40% of the chromium, 85% of the manganese, 75% of the iron, 88% of the cobalt, 68% of the copper, 78% of the zinc, 16% of the selenium, and 48% of the molybdenum (4).

Freezing and canning also decrease nutrient content. Foods are blanched (treated with boiling water or steam) prior to being frozen or canned, and nutrients are destroyed by the heat or lost into the water. Vitamin C, thiamin, and pantothenic acid are extremely vulnerable to heat destruction and, along with riboflavin, to treatment with water. Minerals, including manganese, cobalt, and zinc, tend to be lost into the liquid bathing the food in cans; they nourish only the kitchen drain if thrown away.

Canned or frozen fruits and vegetables can lose some nutrients during storage. The loss depends somewhat on the particular food; frozen broccoli, spinach, cauliflower, and peaches can lose 20% to 50% of their vitamin C content even if stored at −5°F; however, asparagus, beans, and peas can retain over 90% of their vitamin C when frozen for as long as a year (4). The temperature at which canned foods are stored also affects their nutrient content. Canned citrus fruit juice kept at 45°F retains all its vitamin C; but since supermarkets and home pantries are usually kept warmer, some loss of vitamin C does occur. The new open code dating on the labels of cans allows the consumer to determine how long a can has been around and to estimate its vitamin and mineral content. More accurate information is available in books which list the nutrient composition of food.[2] Comparisons can be made of the nutrient content of fresh, canned, dehydrated, and frozen versions of the same food. A comparison makes apparent the nutrient losses due to processing.

Nutrients can also be lost when food is prepared at home. For example:

1. Some people add baking soda to the water in which green vegetables are cooked to help them stay green. It works, but the baking soda makes the vegetables lose considerable amounts of vitamin C and thiamin.

2. The long, slow cooking of meat in a liquid (pot roasting, braising, stewing) causes greater destruction of thiamin than does broiling, roasting, or pan frying. Riboflavin and niacin are also lost into the cooking liquid (or gravy) but can be eaten if the gravy or sauce is served with the meat. (The loss of nutrients as a result of pot roasting or cooking in a slow cooker should not dissuade you from using these cooking methods, especially since they allow the use of leaner cuts of meat. Thiamin is easily obtained from other sources: beans, dairy products, and some vegetables and fruits.)

3. Cooked vegetables and fruits contain fewer nutrients than uncooked food. The nutrient loss is small, however, if the amount of water used is small and the cooking time brief. Steaming and stir-frying maintain the nutrient content better than boiling vigorously in large quantities of water (which are usually discarded).

Steamers are inexpensive and easy to use; they are placed in a pot containing a small amount of water. The pot is covered and the water boiled; the steam from the water cooks the vegetables or fruit. Stir-frying requires only a heavy skillet, a small amount of oil, a wooden spoon, and a quick hand.

Rice and pastas should be cooked in the amount of water called for in the directions on the package; larger amounts of water increase nutrient loss. Rice should not be rinsed after cooking; some nutrients stick to the surface of the cooked grains and can be washed away.

4. Vegetables and fruits cooked with their skins on retain slightly more nutrients than ones that are peeled first. (It is also much easier to remove the skins after the food has been cooked—except for baked potatoes.)

---

[2]*Food Values of Portions Commonly Used* (by C. Church and H. Church, 12th ed., 1975, Lippincott, Philadelphia) is an example.

NATURAL AND ORGANIC FOODS

Foods processed without any chemical preservatives or other additives are called *natural foods*. They used to be found only in health food stores or those which cater to the vegetarian and macrobiotic communities. Certain natural foods, however, have become available in some supermarkets since a national market has been established for them. These products include breads, breakfast cereals, pastas, juices, peanut butter, and crackers.

Natural products are bought for different reasons: some people say that natural products taste better, and this is probably true of the foods made by small local businesses that use traditional ingredients and sell their products quickly. Some people believe that products which take months to mold are closer to plastic than to real food, and they find that idea distasteful. Others are actually afraid of chemical preservatives. Still others like to think that personal care has been put into their foods' preparation. (In fact, the loving care received by many natural foods is dispensed by machines in factories owned by national food processing companies.)

> Natural products have recently been expanded into the "munchie" field. A local macrobiotic food store advertised the following snack foods: brown rice crackers, Koishi rice chips, chips wrapped in seaweed, vegetable chips, bar-B-Q chips, onion and garlic chips, and organic pop corn.

Foods produced without chemical fertilizers, pesticides, and herbicides are called *organic foods*. The term is applied to produce, products made from organic grains (e.g., oatmeal), to nuts, seeds, dried fruit, juice, and meat raised on organic corn and grain. There is no nutritional difference between organically and commercially grown produce, although the former may sometimes be better because it is raised locally and the time between harvest and sale is very short (5).

The consumer has no way of knowing whether a product labeled organic is actually produced without the use of pesticides or chemical fertilizers, since there is only sporadic inspection of farms claiming to raise products organically. There have been unverified anecdotes of "organic farmers" who spray their fields between 1 and 3 a.m. and of organic food store owners who buy produce from supermarkets and sell it as organic. Since organic foods are expensive, the consumer should ascertain, as much as possible, that the food is indeed organically grown. Usually a store acquires a reputation for being honest, and it is worthwhile to check out the store's reputation before purchasing anything.

FOOD ADDITIVES

Many people approach the subject of food additives the way I approach the engine of my car: with fear. Ever since I learned that the car runs because of small gasoline explosions in the engine, I have driven with trepidation. However, since there is no alternative to driving, at least some of the time, I have had to accept assurances that these explosions are perfectly controlled and are of no danger to me or my passengers.

People have no alternative to eating food. Some try to avoid foods that contain additives, although doing so is difficult and time-consuming. Most people grudgingly accept the assurances of scientists and government officials that there is no danger from an additive.

The best way to deal with the problem of food additives is to learn something about them: why they are used, why some are extremely important in food processing and preservation, why others may be of slight or questionable value, and why still others are currently being evaluated for safety. Table 2 lists the general categories and functions of food additives.

The most widely used additives are the preservatives. Food is extremely vulnerable to deterioration. Molds, fungi, and bacteria are always present, awaiting the opportunity to transform edible food into greenish-blue powder, smelly slime, or sour curd. Time and temperature also take their toll. Dried bagels

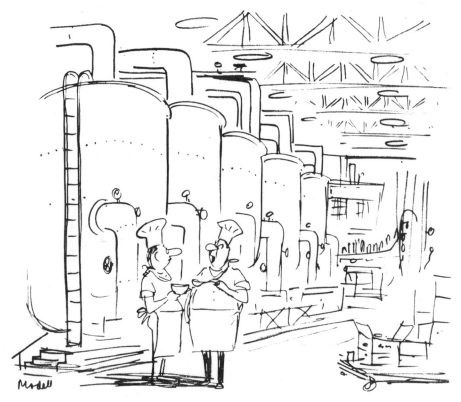

"It needs additives."

(Drawing by Modell; © 1977, The New Yorker Magazine, Inc.)

TABLE 2. *Use of Additives*

Additive	Purpose
Preservatives, antioxidants	Prevent food spoilage caused by microorganisms; prevent rancidity, discoloration
Sequestrants	Bind trace metals to prevent processes resulting in rancidity; prevent minerals from discoloring soft drinks; maintain color in mayonnaise, canned beans, salad dressings, other foods
Humectants	Absorb water and maintain correct "humidity" in foods; used in products such as shredded coconut and marshmallows
Anticaking agents	Ensure free flow of salts and powders such as powdered sugars
Glazing agents	Maintain shiny surfaces on foods
Firming agents	Prevent processed fruits from becoming flabby and mushy; used in pickles, canned peas, apples; also help coagulate milk proteins in manufacture of some cheeses
Foaming agents and foam inhibitors	Keep foods such as whipped cream foaming as they emerge from container; put foam on top of hot chocolate mixes. Inhibitors: prevent foam from interfering with filling of containers such as foam on citrus fruit juice
Stabilizers and thickeners	Give foods a smooth texture; thicken beverages, jams, jellies, ice cream; prevent water from freezing into crystals
Emulsifiers	Keep oil and water mixed, as in salad dressings; prevent fat-containing foods such as chocolate from separating from other ingredients; prevent whitish "bloom" from appearing on chocolate candy; improve texture on baked goods; can replace egg yolks
Acidity and alkalinity agents	Increase or decrease acidity; increase intensity of flavor, improve texture of processed cheese
Leavening agents	Lighten (leaven) baked products
Bleaching and maturing agents	"Whiten" flour and some cheeses; change, or "mature," the texture of flour to improve its baking qualities
Flavors and flavor enhancers	Impart flavors or increase intensity of flavors
Coloring agents	Intensify natural colors or impart new colors
Nutrients	Vitamins, minerals, and protein added to improve nutritional quality of the food or to increase availability of nutrients that are hard to obtain in the diet, such as iron or iodine

useful only as hockey pucks, mushy strawberries, flat whipped cream, limp oatmeal cookies, and powdery garlic cloves are but a few examples. Natural enzymes in food also cause unpleasant though harmless changes in food: the browning of a sliced apple, the pink-brown of a peeled potato (a grated potato turns pink within minutes), black spots on a very ripe banana skin. Man has been fighting these processes for thousands of years. Until recently his weapons were few. He could preserve foods by salting (pork, cod, anchovies), adding large quantities of sugar (jams, jellies), fermentation (sauerkraut, wine), pickling in a vinegar and salt brine (pickles, herring), drying (fruit, beef jerky, fish), smoking (bacon, ham, smoked salmon), cooking, or freezing. Cooking only delayed spoilage (a roast chicken does spoil but not as rapidly as a raw one); and freezing, once the Ice Age was over, was limited to winter or home on the Arctic Circle. Many of these processes are used today to preserve a major portion of our foods. Unfortunately, each process alters the quality of the foods. Pickles are not cucumbers, raisins are not grapes, canned peas do not taste like fresh peas, nor does blueberry jam taste like freshly picked blueberries. Moreover, some forms of processing actually make food temporarily inedible; in order to be consumed, the food must be thawed, soaked, drained, or rinsed. Once these foods are brought back to an edible state, they are again subject to natural deterioration. There is a solution to this problem (other than eating everything as soon as it is thawed, soaked, etc.), and that is to add chemical preservatives to foods so they do not have to undergo freezing, etc. in the first place.

> Cooks have used chemical additives for years. The use of ascorbic acid, in the form of lemon juice, is traditional for preventing apples from turning brown or potatoes from turning pink. Cooks put sugar or egg whites on pie crusts to keep them from becoming too soggy, or add baking soda to keep vegetables green while they are cooking in water.

Most chemical preservatives were developed after the Second World War as part of the new technology of convenience foods. Today the number of highly processed convenience foods is enormous. A glance inside a typical American kitchen would be sure to reveal some of them: breakfast cereals, batter-whipped bread, crackers, instant gravies, dry soups, powdered hot chocolate mix, and margarine. Foods prepared in industrial kitchens may remain uneaten for months. They must be transported to warehouses, supermarkets, and then homes, sometimes with long waits in between. During this time they are vulnerable to many kinds of deterioration; additives are thus used to maintain the safety and quality of the foods.

> Cake mixes contain antioxidants, additives which keep fats and oils from turning rancid. Cake mixes are sometimes used months after they are packaged and would be inedible if antioxidants were not used.
>
> Ice cream forms ice crystals when it is melted and refrozen. Ice cream sold in the supermarket is exposed to many changes in temperature before it reaches the home freezer (especially during a heat wave). Since most consumers prefer a creamy, smooth texture rather than the sharp, tasteless sensation of ice crystals, manufacturers add a seaweed derivative, carrageenin. Carrageenin makes ice cream thicker and prevents formation of ice crystals (6).

Even people who do not buy many highly processed foods have had their shopping habits influenced by the widespread use of preservatives. We expect most fresh foods to remain edible for at least a week and many staple items to stay good for several weeks. Bread should remain soft and free from mold until that last sandwich is made; breakfast cereals are expected to remain crunchy even when the kitchen feels as humid as a jungle in the rainy season; margarine is not supposed to turn rancid. Indeed we are so accustomed to foods remaining fresh that we are horrified when we find a piece of moldy bread or discover milk that has turned sour.

> In the musical, *Fiddler on the Roof,* Tevye, the milkman, goes around the village selling milk and cheese. His products are usually consumed within a few hours, sometimes even minutes. He does not need to add potassium sorbate to his cheese as does the Wisconsin manufacturer of cheddar cheese whose product may not be sold for weeks or months after it leaves the factory.

It is easy to appreciate the time, effort, and money saved by the use of chemical preservatives when we consider how rapidly spoilage occurs in foods to which additives are not or cannot be added. Each time we discard a moldy piece of fruit or discover that the cottage cheese does not smell right, we realize how rapidly food deteriorates. Without additives, we would have to shop twice a day for some foods, and we would have to accept the altered quality of foods preserved by traditional means.

Enormous numbers of chemically derived flavors and colors have been developed by the food industry. Some foods need these additives to replace natural flavors and colors lost during processing. Other foods require the additives because they are made from tasteless, colorless ingredients (or ingredients that impart an unacceptable color or flavor). In these cases the food industry uses additives to make the culinary equivalent of a silk purse from a sow's ear. Food technologists may not start with pig's ears, but the relationship between the raw material and the finished product sometimes seems just as farfetched. For example, such materials as yeast powders, soybean proteins, food starch, whey (a milk protein), peanut flakes, and imitation tomato color may end up as "turkey roll," "bacon," "tomato" sauce, imitation cheese, high-protein breads and rolls, imitation chocolate Bavarian cream pie, instant sour cream sauce, or imitation whipped cream. The list of fabricated food products runs into the thousands, and new ones are constantly being developed to meet real or created needs.

> The predecessor of margarine, oleo, was a white shortening-like substance enclosed in a plastic bag with a capsule of yellow-orange oil. Housewives squeezed the oil from the capsule and kneaded it into the shortening so that after 15 minutes or so of patient pounding the shortening began to resemble, vaguely, "the more expensive spread." The flavor of the oleo was unaffected by its color, but its acceptability was greatly influenced by its appearance.

More recent technology has given us imitation bacon made from soybeans, eggs made with vegetable oil, and fruit drink made from water and sugar; the list of artificially created foods seems endless. These and countless other products are given recognizable identities by coloring and flavoring agents which mimic a natural product. Other products (e.g., grape-flavored chewing gum, cheese- and barbecue-flavored corn chips, fruit-flavored breakfast cereal) are products created from the imagination and technology of food scientists, and contain flavoring and coloring agents to produce a "special effect" the way an artist uses colors to create a painting.

Additives are also used to make technically perfect products. Food starch, for example, is used to thicken runny, soupy, juicy foods such as fruit pie fillings, tomato sauce, gravies, and the flavorings inside doughnuts. Lecithin, which keeps oil (or fat) and water mixed, is found in chocolate candy bars (it prevents chocolate from turning a grayish color), powdered chocolate mixes (it helps them dissolve quickly in water), and the coatings of ice cream sold on a stick (it keeps the chocolate on the ice cream). Lecithin also produces a fluffy texture in breads, doughnuts, cakes, and muffins. [The food additive lecithin contains only about 20% lecithin. Lecithin is a fat-like substance also made in our bodies and is used in the formation of bile salts, cell membranes, lipoproteins, and, indirectly, acetylcholine, a chemical of the nervous system. (Caution: Lecithin food supplements contain between 3 and 30% actual lecithin.)] Other chemical additives prevent dry ingredients from caking or lumping, prevent beverages from becoming cloudy or discoloring, or keep chewy foods chewy and soft foods soft.

As mentioned above, vitamins and minerals are also added to foods to replace those lost during food processing or to confer some nutritional value to a food made from nutritionally empty ingredients.

CONTROVERSIAL ADDITIVES

Food additives seem to be receiving the type of publicity usually associated with crooked politicians, oil spills, and winter weather reports. After reading some accounts of the dangers of food additives, a person might wonder whether he would be safer eating the newsprint than the food. We are understandably puzzled when an additive is still in food after reading that it causes tumors in rats, genetic changes in bacteria, and untimely deaths in mice. Conversely, should an additive be associated with some harmful effect in laboratory animals but seemingly irreplaceable in our food supply, we tend to ask ourselves whether the conditions under which the additive was tested apply to our own eating; we sometimes prefer to retain the ingredient in our food if we arrive at satisfactory answers. (The ban against saccharin is an example of this.) We also wonder why, after 80 years or more of use in our food supply, the safety of certain food additives is being investigated. For example, oil of nutmeg and caffeine are now being evaluated to determine their safety for human consumption; yet both these foodstuffs have been consumed for hundreds of years.

To put our concerns and bewilderment into perspective, we must look at the recent history of food additive regulations and at current methods of evaluating safety. In 1958 a law was passed (the Food Additives Amendment to the Food, Drug, and Cosmetic Act of 1938) preventing the use of new food additives unless they passed certain standards. There had to be evidence of their usefulness and their harmlessness. Furthermore, additives could not be used if they disguised unsafe processing techniques or could lead the shopper to believe that the quality of the food was better than it actually was. For example, artificial colors or flavors could not be used to mask spoiled, stale, or inferior products. (Before these regulations came into effect, many deceptive practices were used, such as putting chalk into flour to whiten it.) Additives already in common use (e.g., nutmeg) were exempted from these regulations and put on a list of additives "generally recognized as safe" (GRAS). Not all food additives in use before 1958 were automatically put on the GRAS list; flavoring substances (which number over 1,200) were turned over to the Flavor and Extract Manufacturers' Association (FEMA) for separate review. Those meeting FEMA's safety standards were classified as FEMA compounds and listed in a government publication called the *Code of Federal Regulations.* (Some of the substances include flavors such as artificial pot roast, watermelon, and cream cheese.)

In 1969 the President ordered a full-scale appraisal of all substances on the GRAS list (8). This occured after the artificial sweetener cyclamate had been removed from the GRAS list because it had been shown to cause cancer in laboratory animals. A committee of scientists (each of whom was well known for his own research) was formed to review and evaluate all of the scientific studies available on the safety of substances found on the GRAS list. The committee, known as SCOGS (Select Committee on GRAS Substances), began its work in 1972. The members read, discuss and evaluate the scientific literature and hold meetings to obtain more information from other scientists, the food industry, and consumer groups.

> Food additives are tested in several ways to determine their safety. They are given in very high doses to test animals in order to determine their lethality as well as the types of change in the organs and tissues such high doses are apt to produce. Lower doses of the additives are also administered to test animals over their lifetimes to obtain information on their safety when consumed continually. (The doses used, although too low to kill the animal, are still higher than that normally consumed by the human on a daily basis.) They are also given to pregnant animals to measure the effect of the additive on fetal development. The offspring are then continued on the dose so the effect of the additive on both fetal and adult life is demonstrated. Some additives have been "fed" to bacteria; i.e., they have been put into the medium in which bacteria grow to test the ability of the substances to cause mutations. Since bacteria reproduce very rapidly, genetic mutations can be detected within a few days.

The results of these studies should establish the safety of a food additive. If there is insufficient evidence, however, the committee can recommend further testing of the additive being evaluated. While the new tests are carried out, the use of the additive is limited to products in which it is already found. It cannot be used in new products or recipes. Should an additive fail to meet the committee's criteria for safety (i.e., if reliable scientific studies show that it causes tumors, fetal malformations, or genetic changes), the additive is dropped from the GRAS list.

The recommendations of the GRAS committee are implemented by the FDA. The decision of the FDA to allow additives to remain in the food supply is governed by the Delaney Clause. This is a law, inserted in the 1958 Food Amendment Act, which states that "no additive shall be deemed to be safe if it is found to induce cancer when ingested by man or animals." This means that an additive which is safe in doses normally consumed by man must be removed from the food supply if excessively large doses cause cancer in laboratory animals. The scientific community and the food industry have criticised the Delaney Clause, and recently, in the case of saccharin, so has the public. The Clause does not allow substances to remain in food even if they are shown to be harmless in doses equivalent to those normally consumed by humans over a lifetime.

Some scientists believe that giving large doses of a chemical and showing that it causes cancer is not irrefutable evidence that taking small doses of the same chemical over a lifetime will also cause cancer. They believe that the body may handle high and low doses of the same substance differently (even high doses of water can be toxic). The following excerpt humorously describes the belief that the safety of food additives cannot be determined by testing extremely large doses on experimental animals.

> Alice asks the Mad Hatter and March Hare if she can eat some ham. "No, No," cried the March Hare. "Bad, bad," yelled the Mad Hatter. "Belch" went the Dormouse. The Hatter tells her: "We've concluded from tests that these foods are bad for you." When she asks what kind of tests, Alice is told: "We stuff as much food as possible into the Dormouse...." "And," continued the Hatter, "if he belches after we've stuffed him full, we know the food is bad." They demonstrate by stuffing a large platter of food into the Dormouse and the Hatter tells Alice to listen. The inevitable belch which follows is cited as evidence that the food was bad. But Alice objects: "You gave him so much food. Why don't you feed him only a reasonable amount?" "Because," replied the Hatter, "then he wouldn't belch." "But," cried Alice, "wouldn't anyone belch like that if you made them eat so much food?" "How should we know," said the Hatter, "we haven't tried" (8a).

There are many scientists who feel that all substances shown to be carcinogenic, regardless of the doses used in testing, should be removed from the food supply. Until recently the FDA was compelled to abide by the Delaney Clause, and so they removed any additive that caused cancer in experimental animals, regardless of the dose used.

Recent legislative action in response to the findings that saccharin causes cancer in laboratory animals may result in a more flexible law. Saccharin has been in our food supply for more than 80 years, but during the spring of 1977 it was about to be eliminated from food entirely. Saccharin, fed in doses equal to about 5% of the total food intake, had caused bladder tumors in 3 out of 100 test rats. Their offspring were given the same dose of saccharin, first as fetuses (their mothers ate it) and then throughout development and adult life. Fourteen of the 100 rats in this group developed bladder tumors. In accordance with the Delaney Clause, the FDA announced that saccharin would be banned. This ban produced enormous public interest; people wanted to keep saccharin. Pressure was brought to bear on Congress to prevent the FDA from removing this additive. The Delaney Clause was circumvented by a Congressional bill that postponed the FDA ban for 18 months, and work was immediately begun on another bill allowing saccharin to be sold with a label warning that it causes cancer in laboratory animals. This warning is now put on vending machines that dispense soft drinks and on the containers themselves.

The ability of rat studies to predict if saccharin is carcinogenic in humans was recently questioned as a result of a study on the incidence of bladder cancer. Over 500 patients with this type of cancer were questioned to learn about their patterns of saccharin and cyclamate consumption. Their intake of these non-nutritive sweeteners was compared with control subjects who were matched in number, age, occupation, sex and habits such as smoking. No difference in the consumption of saccharin or cyclamates was found among the two groups even though one had developed the type of cancer associated with saccharin consumption by experimental animals (8b).

The response to the saccharin ban may ultimately bring about replacement of the Delaney Clause with a law requiring that the evaluation of a food additive include its benefits as well as its dangers. Fortunately, few food additives would require this type of evaluation since safe substitutes can be found for many of them.

> Saccharin cannot be replaced at present because no other nonnutritive sweetener is available for use in diet foods, foods for diabetics, sugarless gums, toothpaste flavorings, and flavorings and coatings for medicines. As soon as a substitute which meets the FDA safety standards is found, saccharin will most likely be removed from the food supply. A new sweetener, aspartame, is going through the final stages of testing, and there is good reason to believe that it might replace saccharin for certain uses (9). However, its instability in solution limits its use in canned foods, bottled beverages, toothpaste, and other water-containing preparations.

Should we eat foods that contain saccharin? Two aspects of the problem should be considered. The first is the alleged benefits from saccharin use: It decreases, for some eaters, the consumption of sugar and thus cuts down on calorie intake; it allows diabetics to eat sweet-flavored foods; it permits gum chewing without inducing cavities; it prevents the crying and anguish when parents must convince their children to take bitter medicine, and it makes toothpaste pleasant enough so that toothbrushing is enjoyed by children. The second aspect concerns the amount of saccharin consumed. A much quoted German–Swiss physician, Paracelsus (first known as Theophratus Bombastus Von Hohenheim), suggested that the "dose makes the poison." Moderation in the consumption of anything, be it saccharin or garlic, is always wise. Limiting saccharin consumption to moderate amounts can be done by considering the reasons for eating saccharin-flavored beverages and foods. If a person adds saccharin instead of sugar to his coffee to reduce caloric intake, especially if he is on a diet, then saccharin is probably beneficial to his diet. Unless he consumes 25 cups of coffee a day, he is actually ingesting relatively small amounts of this artificial sweetener. However, if he adds the saccharin to his coffee, not to cut down on the total amount of calories in his diet but to "save the calories" so he can eat a calorie-laden dessert or snack without guilt, he is abusing his right to use the additive. A teaspoon of sugar contains only 16 calories, a piece of apple pie over 300. The mathematics of this use of saccharin to save calories do not add up to a decrease in calorie intake. In this case, the use of saccharin is unnecessary.

The review of the GRAS list of additives has raised public controversy about the safety of some other well-known, long-used substances: BHA, BHT, sodium nitrite, and sodium nitrate.

BHT and BHA (butylated hydroxytoluene and butylated hydroxyanisole) are preservatives that prevent foods from becoming rancid. They are put into any food which contains butter, oil, fat, margarine, or fatty acids; some examples are ready-to-eat cereals, potato chips, candy; processed foods containing sour cream, butter, margarine, lard, or oil; frozen dairy products such as whipped cream; products containing nuts; cake mixes; frozen waffles; and countless others.

The SCOGS' recent studies on the safety of BHA and BHT indicate that these substances may be harmful to rats (the laboratory animals in which BHA and BHT were tested). The liver of the rat, however, does not handle BHT and BHA in the same way that the human liver does, and the results of this research may not be applicable to humans. The SCOGS recommended that additional research be carried out. The safety of BHA and BHT is sufficiently assured to allow these additives to remain in foods for the present. (Indeed their presence may be beneficial to our health as they prevent the formation of substances called free radicals, which have been shown to cause damage to cell membranes. These free radicals, which form when foods become rancid, are now being studied for their possible toxic effects in humans.)

Sodium nitrate and sodium nitrite are additives used to protect cured and smoked foods against contamination by a deadly bacterium, *Clostridium botulinum.* These bacteria grow in an environment which contains little or no oxygen and have been found in improperly prepared canned foods and under-processed vacuum-packed foods (canned ham, for example); they may also be able to thrive in the interior parts of smoked or cured meats and fish (where there is little or no oxygen). Since the presence of the bacteria and the toxin they produce cause no detectable change in the appearance, taste, or odor of food, we have no way of knowing whether a food is contaminated with the bacteria. The toxin is powerful and deadly, and hence food processors and the U.S. Department of Agriculture (USDA) have been very concerned about preventing the growth of this bacterium. However, during the past few years evidence has been accumulating which indicates that the preservatives sodium nitrate and nitrite, which have been protecting us against the growth of this bacteria, may be harmful themselves.

Nitrates and nitrites can combine with substances called amines (compounds similar to amino acids in structure) to form nitrosamines. Some nitrosamines have been shown to cause cancer in laboratory animals. Although our own bodies apparently make nitrosamines in the stomach from nitrates and nitrites in foods,[3]

---

[3]Nitrates and nitrites are natural food constituents and are found in vegetables, fruits, dairy products, bread and water. More than 80% of the nitrite entering our stomachs comes from saliva (12); about 20% comes from nitrites in cured meats. However, nitrites *per se* have recently been shown to cause tumors in laboratory animals.

the preformed nitrosamines (those formed in foods before they are eaten) are considered more carcinogenic (10). Cooking foods which contain nitrites increases the concentration of nitrosamines. [Cured meat products such as bacon contain detectable levels of nitrosamines when heated to 360°F (11) for 6 minutes or more.] Consequently the USDA is requiring bacon manufacturers to decrease the amount of nitrite used in processing and to add sodium ascorbate or sodium erythorbate, substances that block nitrosamine formation. [An alternative may be buying precooked microwaved bacon. Cooking bacon by microwave protects it from *C. botulinum* growth, and thus the nitrite content can be reduced substantially (11).]

> There is also some evidence that another substance, potassium sorbate, may be as effective as nitrite in reducing the growth of the botulism organism, and its addition to cured meats would allow nitrite concentration to be reduced further.

Some types of cured foods contain nitrates and nitrites because these additives confer a red color, as well as a flavor and consistency, to these products. Thus frankfurters, luncheon meats, salami, and sausage contain nitrites for their flavor and color-producing qualities, not because they are needed to prevent botulism. As long as these products are refrigerated at a temperature below 40°F at all times, they can be made without these preservatives. It is easy to recognize a frankfurter made without nitrates or nitrites; it is the color of cooked meat —gray.

Despite the evidence that nitrosamines can cause cancer in laboratory animals, there is no evidence at present that *any* human cancer has resulted from nitrosamines in foods (12). Certainly we should not stop eating the foods that naturally contain nitrites; doing so would result in eliminating many important nutrients from our diet. More and more cured foods will be processed without added nitrites, or with reduced levels, so it will be possible to eat hot dogs or canned ham and consume only small amounts of these additives. As with the consumption of other additives, moderation is the wisest course. If cured meats made without nitrates and nitrites are available, eating them rather than the same foods made with nitrites is a sensible way of reducing nitrite consumption. (Check labels, some manufacturers are coloring nonnitrite-containing meats with beet juice or other red colors.)

As consumer interest grows in consuming nitrite-free foods, more manu-facturers will voluntarily eliminate nitrites from foods if doing so does not result in any danger from the botulism organism.

Monosodium glutamate (MSG) is an additive that brings out flavors already present in foods. It has attained some notoriety, especially among eaters of Chinese food. About 10 years ago a report in the *New England Journal of Medicine* described three ill effects felt by patrons of Chinese restaurants (13). These symptoms, together called Chinese restaurant syndrome, were sensations of burning, tightness, and pressure (or numbness) in the face, chest, or neck. They began within 5 minutes after eating and persisted for 2 to 3 hours. It was later shown in clinical tests that certain people fed MSG, a common ingredient in Chinese cooking, experienced these symptoms (14).

As people learned about Chinese restaurant syndrome, they naturally tended to assume that MSG was responsible for other kinds of discomfort they felt after eating in Chinese restaurants. [It is extremely common for people to feel some discomfort after eating away from home (15).] Even articles in popular publications reported symptoms such as headache, dizziness, weakness, and sweating to be part of the Chinese restaurant syndrome and caused by MSG. In fact, these symptoms probably have different causes; only burning, tightness, and pressure have, in scientific studies, been associated with MSG, and people studying Chinese restaurant syndrome prefer to limit its definition to those three symptoms.

> Efforts to confirm even these limited effects of MSG have not always been successful. In one set of tests, for example, some people were given beef broth containing MSG, and others were given broth without the additive; no one was told what his broth contained. Both groups of people reported symptoms after drinking the broth, regardless of its MSG content (16). In another study it was necessary to give volunteers a 2% solution of MSG (considerably more than most people would eat at one time) in order to produce any effect. However, about 25% of the subjects did experience symptoms characteristic of Chinese restaurant syndrome (17).

Some people, of course, may be especially sensitive to MSG, as others are to garlic, green peppers, or chocolate. A variety of processed foods contain it, and people who believe they are sensitive to MSG should read labels. Restaurants vary in their use of MSG; it might be worthwhile for those who often have indigestion after eating out to buy some MSG (it is sold in the spice section of the supermarket, although sometimes it is available only under the Accent trade name) and test a little on themselves to see if it is the culprit.

In 1969 a scientist injected extremely large quantities of MSG into newborn mice (18) and into a premature newborn monkey (19). He reported evidence of brain damage and thus opened up another area of uncertainty concerning the use of MSG. Similar experiments carried out on chicks and rabbits produced the same results (20). However, when the same amounts of MSG were *fed* rather than injected into infant monkeys, no damage to the brain was found (21, 22). Therefore many scientists have questioned whether results obtained by *injecting* a food additive rather than by *feeding* it are really useful in evaluating the additive's safety. Moreover, research is continuing on how MSG causes brain damage when injected, and whether the same effect could be produced by injecting large quantities of other substances such as salt.

Caffeine is another controversial substance. It occurs naturally in coffee and cocoa; and a similar compound, theophylline, is found in tea. Caffeine is also added to cola drinks and to cold and pain medications. (American parents usually try to delay their children's coffee drinking with the warning, "Coffee will stunt your growth!" but this statement has never been verified. Countries such as France where coffee drinking is common among the young do not seem to have a disproportionate share of short people.)

However, caffeine and theophylline do have some definite effects; they increase alertness, decrease drowsiness and fatigue, and are particularly good in preventing attention lapses in night drivers. Caffeine is addictive. People accustomed to drinking several cups of coffee a day can get severe headaches or become sleepy or irritable if denied coffee for a day or two. Conversely, those who drink relatively little coffee sometimes have difficulty falling asleep if they drink coffee during the evening. People who have this problem should look for caffeine on the label of cold or pain medications taken at bedtime. (Habitual coffee drinkers are usually unaffected.)

In a recent study caffeine was shown to increase blood pressure, the secretion of certain hormones such as epinephrine (adrenaline), and the output of urine, and to change the heart rate in noncoffee drinkers who were given a dose of caffeine equal to that found in three cups of coffee (23). The effect of caffeine on these bodily functions in habitual coffee drinkers has not yet been tested. However, the scientists who conducted this study suggest that people who have a tendency toward high blood pressure (hypertension) might be especially susceptible to the effects of caffeine.

> At one time coffee was thought to be related to heart attacks. Fortunately, further study showed that coffee drinking itself did not increase the risk of heart attack; rather, it was the smoking which usually accompanied coffee drinking that was responsible (24).

An excessive amount of caffeine ("excessive" amounts vary from one person to the next) can cause nervousness, irritability, insomnia, flushing, and gastrointestinal disturbance. Children who consume excessive amounts of soft drinks containing caffeine may experience symptoms similar to those felt by an adult who drinks too many cups of coffee. However, children who drink 10 or 12 cans of soda daily will have other problems as well, such as the effects of sugar on their teeth or the absence of nutrients they would be getting in milk or juice. Children should not be encouraged to drink large amounts of soda regardless of its caffeine content; the small amount of caffeine in a single can of soda is not dangerous, however. [It is about the same as the caffeine in a cup of cocoa. Five ounces of a cola drink contains 50 milligrams of caffeine; a chocolate bar contains 25 milligrams (25).]

Coffee, like other beverages and foods, should be taken in moderation. The appropriate amount varies; 12 cups a day may be normal for one person; 12 cups a year for another. Most habitual coffee, tea, or cola consumers know their own limitations and can recognize when they are drinking too much.

ADDITIVES AND HYPERKINESIS

Certain types of food additives may be related to hyperkinesis, or hyperactivity. Many parents call their normal, highly active children hyperactive, but in medical teminology a hyperactive (hyperkinetic) child is one with a serious behavioral disorder. Hyperactive children are usually males of elementary school age; they have learning difficulties, short attention span, and extreme restlessness, and their emotions change rapidly (26). No one knows what causes this disorder, although it is generally believed that the same symptoms may have many different causes. Until recently the only effective treatment for hyperkinesis was medication. Now a new dietary treatment is being studied.

Allergist Dr. Ben Feingold found that some hyperactive children got better when placed on what he called an "elimination diet" (27), i.e., a diet which eliminates all synthetic colors, flavors, and salicylates. (The active compound in aspirin is a salicylate; salicylates also occur naturally in oranges, apples, plums, peaches, berries, tomatoes, apricots, cucumbers, and almonds.)

The American Academy of Pediatrics decided to check Dr. Feingold's reports with a series of studies (28). In one such study, hyperactive children ate two special diets, each for several weeks. One was the Feingold diet; the other was a normal diet but with certain foods arbitrarily omitted so the children's parents and teachers would think it also was therapeutic. The teachers reported a significant improvement in the behavior of the children eating the Feingold diet. Parents also noted an improvement, but some reported improvement with the other diet as well (28).

Additional studies were done to test whether children on the Feingold diet would become more hyperactive if (unknown to them, their parents, and teachers) they were given food colors to eat. (The colors were concealed in a chocolate bar developed for this purpose by a food company). This was done with a group of children whose parents and teachers thought their behavior had improved on the Feingold diet. Unexpectedly, only one child became more hyperactive. The other children were not affected. In another study, children were given a test to see if their attention span was changed by eating these additives after they had been on the Feingold diet for several weeks. They did not do as well on the test as they had before eating the additives; however, the effect lasted only about 2 hours (29).

The conclusion thus far is that very few hyperactive children are clearly better when put on a Feingold diet, but that there are some who, for unknown reasons, are sensitive to food additives. More studies are under way to see if the age of a child influences his response to this elimination diet (29). Parents of hyperactive children should seek the advice of their pediatrician when deciding whether to try the diet; the American Academy of Pediatrics cautions that the diet should be tried only under medical supervision. A list of references on diet and hyperactivity appears at the end of the chapter under *Recommended Reading*.

Should we eliminate all additive-containing foods from the diet? Clearly the answer is "no" based on the scientific evidence attesting to the safety of most additives in our food supply. As pointed out in the preceding section, a sensible response to evidence indicating that a few additives (nitrites, BHT, saccharin) are toxic in laboratory animals is to reduce consumption of them to moderate or low amounts. Some people feel strongly about not eating foods which contain additives and so change their eating style to avoid them. However, avoiding additive-containing foods imposes a hardship since it eliminates an enormous variety of foods for home consumption and indeed restricts eating out to natural-food restaurants. This hardship is unnecessary since moderate consumption of additives has not been shown to be dangerous.

It is possible to reduce the *amount* of additives consumed without drastically changing our way of eating. To do this we must first learn which types of food that contain additives are eaten regularly. This takes only a few minutes. Look around the kitchen and note the foods that contain additives. They fall into three categories: staples, sporadic necessities, and dispensables. Decide which foods fit into the *staple* category. These are foods that are consumed regularly and are unlikely to be purchased without additives or made at home. Such foods may be bread, breakfast cereals, soups, condiments, crackers, pancake syrup, margarine, spices, some cheeses, fruit drinks. Then decide which foods fit into the second category, *sporadic necessities.* These are foods that are kept around the kitchen for emergencies (e.g., a spare cake mix in case you have to make 50 cupcakes at the last minute for the PTA), entertaining, special treats, or holiday or religious celebrations. Finally, decide which foods belong in the third category: *dispensables.* These foods are purchased because they are convenient, fun to eat, or represent a new way of making ordinary entrees interesting. Many of the foods in this category can be eliminated without causing a substantial increase in the work of food preparation or its cost. For example:

1. Chocolate drinks can be replaced by adding cocoa to fresh or powdered milk (or chocolate syrup, which contains a few additives but considerably less than the instant chocolate drink mixes).

2. Instant soups, which contain primarily additives can be replaced by canned soups or dried soups (these take 20 minutes to cook). The long-cooking dried soups do contain some additives but fewer than the instant variety.

3. A box of dinner components such as macaroni and cheese or spaghetti and sauce can be made by buying the components separately. Doing this reduces the amount of additives (as well as the cost).

4. Extenders for hamburger meat, which are made out of soy cereal and spices, can be replaced by buying high-protein baby cereal and adding the spices yourself. (The baby cereal costs considerably less and is additive-free.)

5. Powdered fruit drinks can be replaced by fruit, fruit juice, water, or milk.

6. Bread crumbs can be made within seconds in a blender; bread can be oven-dried and used instead of crackers; stuffing requires only stale bread, an egg, broth, celery, and spices (they do not have to come out of a box); tomato sauce can be made from a can of tomato puree and spices; frankfurters and beans can be combined in your own kitchen.

To find ways of replacing highly processed additive-dense foods with additive-free food, read the label and see what the food manufacturer put into the food. Buy those ingredients (many, such as spices or cocoa, will keep for months) and assemble the dish yourself. These suggestions should produce a decrease in the amount of additives in one's diet without causing too much trouble or inconvenience.

COMMENT

Hunting and gathering food in the modern supermarket can produce a nutritionally complete and safe diet. However, as this chapter has shown, food gathering must not be a haphazard process. Just as primitive man could not casually bring to his cave any food he stumbled across without subjecting his family to the hazards of poisonous or nutritionally poor foods, the modern food gatherer cannot throw foods into a shopping cart without considering their nutritional value. He is more fortunate than his ancient ancestor because he does not have to worry about the immediate safety of his foods. Research and government regulations assure him that, unlike primitive man, he will not die after a mouthful of supper; even substances that are possibly harmful would have to be consumed in large quantities over long periods of time to produce adverse effects. Unlike primitive man, who often faced the risk of being eaten while attempting to find something to eat, the modern shopper faces only the hazard of being hit by a runaway shopping cart.

REFERENCES

1. National Nutrition Consortium, with Deutsch, R. (1975): *Nutrition Labeling, How It Can Work for You.* National Nutrition Consortium, Bethesda.
2. Development aids. *Food Products Dev.,* 11:52, 1977.
3. Pepperoni Pizza, A & P Company, Montvale, New York.
4. Nesheim, R. (1974): Nutrient changes in food processing: A current review. *Fed. Proc.,* 33:2267.
5. Margolius, S. (1973): *Health Foods: Facts and Fakes.* Walker Publishing, New York.
6. Kermode, G.O. (1972): Food additives. *Sci. Am.,* 226:15.
7. Hopkins, H. (1977): Food additives: Double check on safety. *FDA Consumer,* June: 8.
8. Select Committee on GRAS Substances (1977): Evaluation of health aspects of GRAS food ingredients: Lessons learned and questions unanswered. *Fed. Proc.,* 37:2525.
8a. Sayer, M. (1978): Alice in Wonderland, D.C. *Food Products Dev.,* 12:17.
8b. Kessler, I. and Clark, J. (1978): Saccharin, cyclamate and human bladder cancer. *JAMA,* 240:349.
9. Culliton, B. (1977): Fight over the proposed saccharin ban will not be settled for months. *Science,* 196:276.
10. Jukes, T. (1977): Current concepts in nutrition. *N. Engl. J. Med.,* 297:427.
11. Mattson, P. (1978): Bacon precooked by microwaves offers the potential of lowering nitrosamine levels, *Food Products Dev.,* 12:47.
12. Editorial staff (1978): CAST weighs risks and benefits of using nitrite in cured meats. *Food Products Dev.,* 12:89.
13. Kwok, R.H.M. (1968): Chinese-restaurant syndrome. *N. Engl. J. Med.,* 278:796.
14. Amos, M., Leavitt, N.R., Marmorek, L., and Wolschina, S.B. (1969): Sincib, syn: Accent on glutamate. *N. Engl. J. Med.,* 279:105.
15. Kerr, G., Wu-Lee, M., El-Lozy, M., McGandy, S., and Stare, F. (1977): Objectivity of food-symptomatology surveys. *Am. Diet. Assoc.,* 71:263.
16. Morselli, P.L., and Garattini, S. (1970): Monosodium glutamate and the Chinese restaurant syndrome. *Nature (Lond),* 227:661.

17. Kenney, R.A. (1979): Placebo-controlled studies of human reaction to oral monosodium L-glutamate. In: Glutamic Acid: *Advances in Biochemistry and Physiology,* edited by L.J. Filer, Jr., S. Garattini, M.R. Kare, W.A. Reynolds, and R.J. Wurtman. Raven Press, New York *(in press).*
18. Olney, J. (1969): Brain lesions, obesity, and other disturbances in mice treated with monosodium glutamate. *Science,* 164:719.
19. Olney, J., and Sharpe, L. (1969): Brain lesions in an infant rhesus monkey treated with monosodium glutamate. *Science,* 166:386.
20. Olney, J., Ho, O., Rhee, V., and DeGubareff, T. (1973): Neurotoxic effects of glutamate. *N. Engl. J. Med.,* 289:1374.
21. Reynolds, W.A., Filer, L.J., and Pitkin, R.M. (1971): Monosodium glutamate: Absence of hypothalamic lesions after ingestion by newborn primates. *Science,* 172:1342.
22. Stegink, L., Reynolds, W.A., Filer, L.J., Pitkin, R.M., Boaz, D., and Brummel, M. (1975): Monosodium glutamate metabolism in the neonatal monkey. *Am. J. Physiol.,* 229:246.
23. Robertson, D., Frolich, J., Carr, R., Watson, J., Hollifield, J., Shand, D., and Oates, J. (1978): Effects of caffeine on plasma renin activity, catecholamines, and blood pressure. *N. Engl. J. Med.,* 298:181.
24. Yano, K., Rhoads, G., and Kagan, A. (1977): Coffee, alcohol, and risk of coronary heart disease among Japanese men living in Hawaii. *N. Engl. J. Med.,* 289:405.
25. Stephenson, P. (1977): Physiologic and psychotropic effects of caffeine on man. *J. Am. Diet. Assoc.,* 71:240.
26. Lucas, B., and Sells, C. (1977): Nutrient intake and stimulant drugs in hyperactive children. *J. Am. Diet. Assoc.,* 70:373.
27. Feingold, B. (1974): *Why Your Child is Hyperactive.* Random House, New York.
28. Harley, J.P., Tomasi, L., Ray, R., Eichman, P., Matthews, C., Chun, R., Traisman, E., and Cleeland, C. (1977): *An Experimental Evaluation of Hyperactivity and Food Additives, Phase I.* University of Wisconsin, Madison, Wis.
29. Lipton, M., Wender, E., and The National Advisory Committee on Hyperkinesis and Food Additives (1977): *Statement Summarizing Research Findings on the Issues of the Relationship between Food-Additive-Free Diets and Hyperkinesis in Children.* Nutrition Foundation, New York.

RECOMMENDED READING: Hyperkinesis and Diet

1. Conners, C.K., Goyette, C.H., Southwick, D., Lees, J., and Andrulonis, P. (1976): Food additives and hyperkinesis: A controlled double-blind experiment. *Pediatrics,* 58:154.
2. Diet and hyperactivity: any connection? *Nutr. Rev.,* 34:151.
3. Feingold, B.F. (1973): Food additives and child development. *Hosp. Pract.,* October: 11.
4. Feingold, B.F. (1975): Hyperkinesis and learning disabilities linked to artificial food flavors and colors. *Am. J. Nursing,* 75:797.
5. Feingold, B. (1976): Hyperkinesis and learning disabilities linked to the ingestion of artificial food colors and flavors. *J. Learning Disabil.,* 9:551.
6. First report of the preliminary findings and recommendations of the intragency Collaborative Group on Hyperkinesis. Report submitted to the Assistant Secretary for Health, U.S. Dept. of Health, Education and Welfare, Washington, D.C., January, 1976.
7. Harley, J.P., and Matthews, C. (1978): *The Feingold Hypothesis: Current Studies, Contemporary Nutrition,* Vol. 3, edited by A.E. Sloan. Nutrition Dept., General Mills, Minneapolis.
8. Harley, J.P., Tomasi, L., Ray, R., Eichman, P., Matthews, C., Chun, R., Traisman, E., and Cleeland, C. (1977): *An Experimental Evaluation of Hyperactivity and Food Additives, Phase I.* University of Wisconsin, Madison, Wis.
9. Larkin, T. (1977): Food additives and hyperactive children. *FDA Consumer,* March:19.
10. New Clinical Drug Evaluation Unit Program. *Intercom,* 7:1, 1977.
11. Palmer, S., Rapoport, J.L., and Quinn, P.O. (1975): Food additives and hyperactivity: A comparison of food additives in the diets of normal and hyperactive boys. *Clin. Pediatr.,* 14:59.
12. Spring, C., and Sandoval, J. (1976): Food additives and hyperkinesis: A critical evaluation of the evidence. *J. Learning Disabil.,* 9:560.
13. The National Advisory Committee on Hyperkinesis and Food Additives (1975): *Recommen-*

dations for Conducting Research on the Topic of Food Additives and Hyperactivity Made To the Nutrition Foundation. Nutrition Foundation, New York.

14. Williams, J.I., Cram D.M., Tausig, F.T., and Webster, E. (1976): *Determining the Relative Effectiveness of Dietary and Drug Management of Hyperkinesis: A Preliminary Report of Findings.* Health Care Research Unit, University of Western Ontario, Canada.

4 THE OVEREATER: Causes and Cures

Many people in the United States weigh too much. A casual body count at a beach, ball game, or shopping mall confirms studies which show that 30% of our entire population and 50% of those over 65 are overweight. People who exceed their ideal weight by more than 10% to 20% (144 pounds rather than 120 pounds, for example) are called overweight; those whose weight exceeds 20% of their ideal weight are termed obese.

People gain and keep on excess weight for many reasons. The only characteristic common to all overweight people is that they eat and drink more calories than their bodies need. These excess calories are stored as fat. (When a person has stored 3,500 extra calories, he will be a pound heavier.)

> A calorie is a unit of energy. When food has been digested and absorbed, the body's cells convert the chemical energy in the molecules of food into energy-containing compounds that are used by the cells to stay alive and to carry out their particular tasks. Children and adolescents need calories for growth as well. The body also uses energy derived from food as fuel for physical activity. Many people believe that calories are needed *only* for physical activity and feel guilty about eating if they have not exercised. This is wrong; the body needs some energy all the time to carry out the enormous number of chemical activities in the cells which keep us alive. The body stops using calories only when it stops permanently.
>
> All foods contain calories; the number of calories in a food depends on its protein, fat, carbohydrate, and water content. Protein and carbohydrate each contains 4 calories per gram (there are about 28 grams in an ounce), and fat contains about 9 calories per gram. Water contains no calories, which is why vegetables and fruits that have a high water content contain so few calories per gram.

Weight gain occurs over many months if the number of extra calories eaten each day is small (e.g., the equivalent of an apple or a handful of peanuts). (A person can easily gain 100 pounds over a 20-year span—about 5 pounds a year.) Weight can also be gained in spurts. A period of fairly rapid gain can be followed by a period of stability, which may or may not be followed by additional gain.

> A sudden weight gain after a weekend of gustatory indulgence does not usually mean that one has eaten 6,000 or 7,000 extra calories. Often those extra pounds noted on Monday morning are due to the weight of food still in the intestine and to water retention, especially if the food was high in salt content. However, if the feasting continues all week and every week, eventually those Monday pounds will become fat.

The basic cause of weight gain is a *style* of eating that provides more calories than are needed. The excess calories can come packaged in any type of food; weight can be gained whether the surplus is supplied by broccoli or bonbons. Overeaters are not necessarily *big* eaters or people with abnormal eating styles. A secretary who sits at a desk all day may eat considerably less than a woman of similar build who bags groceries all day; yet the secretary may weigh more because she uses fewer calories in physical activity. A member of a cross-country ski team may consume more calories each day than the secretary does in a week; yet because he utilizes so many calories in exercise, his food intake cannot be considered abnormal.

To lose weight, a person must eat fewer calories than his body needs, so that the stored energy (i.e., the fat) will be used up. This principle of weight loss is easy to state; for many people it is difficult, unpleasant, and sometimes impossible to accomplish.

This chapter discusses the more general causes of excess weight gain and the methods currently available to produce weight loss. It is hoped that the overeater and those who know him will gain insight into the complexities of this problem, and learn patience and have sympathy with the processes of its solution.

WHO IS OVERWEIGHT?

There are many ways of telling if a person is overweight. One of the most reliable is to do a skinfold test. A fold of skin on the back of the arm is pinched between the thumb and forefinger or between the points of an instrument called a caliper. The thickness of the pinch measures the amount of subcutaneous fat (fat under the skin). Since subcutaneous fat accounts for about 50% of all fat in the body, charts have been developed that relate this measurement to total body fat and hence to the degree of obesity.

A "do-it-yourself" skin-pinch test can be done. Stand with your arms hanging loosely. (It helps to be assisted in this). Pinch or grasp with the thumb and forefinger a full fold of skin and subcutaneous tissue (but not muscle) from the back of the right upper arm about midway between the shoulder and elbow. The skinfold showing between the fingers should then be measured on a ruler. Table 1 gives the measurements of skinfold thickness which is indicative of obesity.

This method of determining obesity is more reliable than standard height and weight tables. Most tables record the subject's weight in clothes and height with shoes. The weight of the clothing and height of the shoes are then estimated and subtracted from the results. If you weigh yourself in heavier or lighter clothing than that worn by the subjects on whom the tables are based then you may find yourself on the wrong place in the chart. Moreover, little information on body frame is available in these tables except for defining a small, medium, or large frame size based on chest and hip width. Even though such charts are used by doctors, nutritionists, and weight-reducing organizations to determine "ideal" weight, they are so imprecise they can tell an individual only if he is extremely over- or underweight. (And he probably knows the answer to that question already.)

If the charts do not list body frame sizes, they can actually supply erroneous information. One woman comes to mind who had a large frame: she took size 9D

TABLE 1. *Obesity standards in Caucasian Americans*

Age (years)	Minimum triceps, skin-fold thickness indicating obesity (mm)	
	Males	Females
5	12	14
6	12	15
7	13	16
8	14	17
9	15	18
10	16	20
11	17	21
12	18	22
13	18	23
14	17	23
15	16	24
16	15	25
17	14	26
18	15	27
19	15	27
20	16	28
21	17	28
22	18	28
23	18	28
24	19	28
25	20	29
26	20	29
27	21	29
28	22	29
29	22	29
30–50	23	30

From ref. 4, with permission.

shoes and had trouble fitting a woman's wristwatch strap around her wrist. Her weight was ideal for her build, but her physician told her that she was 10 pounds overweight because his chart did not list weight according to skeletal or frame size.

Other methods for determining the fat content of the body are used only in medical research or in clinics dealing with certain types of obesity. They include taking a small plug of tissue from the buttocks and examining it under a microscope to count and measure fat cells;[1] giving a patient radioactive isotopes which measure body water or muscle mass; and measuring the density of the body when submerged under water (fat and lean body masses have different densities, and the fraction of weight contributed by fat can be calculated with this method). Although these methods more precisely define the extent of obesity, they are too costly, time-consuming, and unpleasant to be used by the average person. For some, the visual and clothing tests are the most useful in determining whether one

[1] Adipocytes (fat cells) store lipid (fat) in the body. They are reservoirs (storage sites) of energy. Fat is constantly leaving these cells to be used by other cells as a source of energy, and new fat is constantly being deposited.

④ Vis

④ visual

⑤ Clothing

is indeed getting fat. Looking at yourself in the mirror, trying on clothes not worn for a season, putting on a bathing suit, or going to the store and trying on clothes in a size that used to fit can be as revealing of one's fatness as any chart, skinfold test, or fat cell count. (A few people suffer from the delusion that they are fat when they are actually extremely *under*weight. This is a medically defined syndrome called anorexia nervosa most often seen in teenage girls. Most of us are correct in our appraisals of our bodies, however; if we look fat, our clothes are tight, and we feel fat, then we usually are.)

EATING STYLE OF THE OVERWEIGHT INDIVIDUAL

Overweight people cannot be grouped together as individuals with a common eating history, attitudes toward food, or patterns of weight gain and loss. Each individual, regardless of weight, has a personal style of eating, and this perhaps more than anything else determines the pattern of weight gain or loss. Since this style of eating is made up of myriad personal eating experiences during the past and present, it must be unique for each individual.

Two major categories of overweight people can be identified, however: those who were overweight as children and remained overweight as adults, and those who became overweight during adulthood. There is a third category, the invisible overweight individual. These are people who lost a considerable amount of weight at one time in their lives and now "pass" as lean. However, many never stop believing that they have a problem controlling their weight and continue to think of themselves as a fat person inside a lean body.

Childhood Obesity

Many adults who are overweight, or who are engaged in a constant struggle to keep their weight down, were fat as children. Doctors feel that if causes of childhood obesity can be understood, anticipated, and prevented, much adult obesity can be avoided as well.

Unfortunately, researchers have been unable to agree on the answers to some fundamental questions. Are the causes of obesity environmental, hereditary, or both? Many people who have been overweight since childhood had overweight siblings and parents (1, 2). Did they gain excess weight because of an inherited tendency or because there was too much good food around the house?

This problem has been studied in families that have biological and adopted children. The scientists doing this study assumed that if the tendency toward obesity is inherited, the weights of a biological child and his parent should be more similar than those of the adopted child and the same parent (3). They found that the amount of body fat was similar between parents and children regardless of whether the children were adopted. Hence it is not necessary to be related to someone to eat like him, and this tends to be borne out by the similar shapes of spouses (with the exception of Jack Spratt and his wife), and even dogs and their owners (3).

However, other studies that examined the similarity in weight between identical and fraternal twins indicate that there may be some inheritable traits that affect the amount of food we eat and the way the body uses it for energy (4). Moreover, it has also been argued that we are born with body types which predispose us toward fatness or leanness. These body types, first described by a scientist named Sheldon (5), grouped people into three body types: endomorphs, mesomorphs, and ectomorphs. An endomorph is round and soft; the mesomorph has heavy bones and muscles, and the ectomorph is slight, has relatively long arms and legs, and fine bones. Endomorphs supposedly have a greater tendency to become fat than ectomorphs; mesomorphs are somewhere in the middle. The problem with this theory is that weight gain or loss itself changes body shape or disguises it. Some ectomorphic-looking children (long and lean) become endo-morphic adults because weight gain has rounded their body configurations. (Our poodle has undergone this sort of transformation in recent years.)

Some fairly recent research indicated that obesity in children and adults resulted from obesity during infancy (6). Studies showed that fat cells (adipose tissue) multiply rapidly during infancy and again during adolescence (7). After it was found that some people who had been overweight all their lives had more fat cells than individuals who became fat during young adulthood, some scientists suggested that an overabundance of fat cells formed during infancy or early childhood might predispose a person to obesity throughout life. A fat baby would turn into a fat child, fat teenager, and fat young, middle-aged, and old adult. These grim predictions, which made mothers look with horror at the rolls of fat around their babies' thighs (and thought to be a sign of good health by grandmothers), seemed to be supported by several additional studies that compared the weights of individuals as children and as adults. One report showed that more children who were overweight during their first 6 months of life were overweight as adults than those who had normal weight during those early months (8). However, this report also showed that a child with an overweight parent was more likely to be overweight as an adult. Another study showed that almost half of the children who were obese by age 10 were already obese during their first year of life; the rest had been heavy since age 5 (9). This study also found a strong correlation between obesity in parents and children. The parents of the obese children were "fatter, heavier, shorter, and also older than those of the normal weight children." All this is enough to induce mothers to sign their infants up for diet clubs! A more recent study, however, has come up with contradictory results (10). This one found that very few of the children who were considered overweight during infancy were still overweight by the time they were 5 years old. In fact, most of these heavy infants began to slow down their weight gain during the second 6 months of life. Unfortunately, none of these studies have been carried on long enough to show whether adults who become overweight during middle or old age were also overweight as infants. In the meantime, there is no way of identifying adults of normal weight who were considerably overweight as infants and children. These people are not likely to show up at obesity clinics and to have a plug of tissue removed for fat cell counts. Do they have an excess number of fat cells? No one knows.

Finally, it is important to note that a style of eating develops along with fat cells during infancy and childhood. The family's style of eating might have as long-lasting an influence as the number of fat cells. Hence we cannot be sure whether excess fat cells or a fat-producing style of eating established during childhood causes obesity in adulthood.

Changing a family's eating style may be as difficult as changing the number of their fat cells. Often parents and children do not perceive that their excess weight is due to the way they eat. In many instances there is nothing abnormal about the types of food served, the attitudes of the family toward food, the use of food for family treats or social occasions, or the times and places at which eating occurs. The children and parents may simply eat more food than they need. The servings may be too large, or the number of courses or foods per course excessive; snacking may be frequent and unnecessary; and food may accompany all social events, regardless of whether it is necessary (e.g., eating a candy bar at the movies).

A friend of mine grew up in a family with all of these fat-producing habits. This man was 75 pounds overweight from early adolescence until age 20. After he successfully reduced to a normal weight, he had to learn a new way to eat because the eating style he had learned from his family was appropriate only for weight gain. He had never thought that his family ate excessively; since it was the only way of eating he had known, he had assumed it was normal. Dinner, for example, always consisted of large servings of meat and potatoes or noodles accompanied by two varieties of fresh bread from the bakery, an occasional vegetable like corn, and a salad heavily doused with Russian dressing (the only kind his father would eat). Everyone ate rapidly in order to get another serving of the main course (when I visited the family, I often found dessert served before I had finished my first serving of the main course). They always ate dessert: pie, cake, pudding, or ice cream regardless of whether they were full by the time it was served. Indeed they were sometimes cautioned to "leave room for dessert" if they asked for a third helping of meat. Soda was drunk during the meal. Moreover, portions were always large (a 3-ounce serving of meat was regarded as an appetizer). No one ever used low-calorie vegetables (e.g., cucumbers or celery) to assuage his hunger.

Occasionally, a family member would feel guilt about overeating, usually following consumption of a pound of chocolate, a banana split, or several forays to the buffet table at a wedding reception.

During and after his weight loss, my friend taught himself the caloric value of foods; he learned to fill up on bulky, low-calorie foods at the start of a meal so he would be content with a small serving of the main course; he eliminated most of the foods he loved as a child and never ate an unfamiliar food without first checking its caloric level.

I once asked him when he had last eaten a candy bar. His eyes became slightly moist as he recollected that wonderful pound bar of Hershey's chocolate he had consumed all alone the summer before his diet began. The foods his mother served so often are only a memory. He does not allow himself to eat them now. They have been outgrown and put away, as a child puts away a tricycle when he starts riding a two-wheeler.

Some adults never put away their childhood eating styles. Dieting represents extreme deprivation and unless the individual consciously decides to teach himself a new style of eating, he often reverts to childhood eating patterns as soon as the dieting period ends.

Obesity and lack of physical activity often perpetuate each other in the overweight family. Although children of overweight parents do not invariably spend childhood in a chair, they may have to seek opportunities for physical activity outside the family with friends, at school, and in camps and clubs. If a child becomes considerably heavier than his peers, he is often excluded from their activities or is included only grudgingly (being chosen last for a game of kickball or always holding the jump rope rather than jumping). These children come to think of themselves as unathletic, and when they are old enough for competitive sports choose not to participate because they already "know" they will not make the team. Their parents do not offer encouragement since they fail to perceive physical inactivity as a problem. It then becomes very difficult for these children to change their self-image and act differently from the rest of the family.

> This is clearly illustrated by two families lying on a beach. Each family had several daughters between the ages of 9 and 15. One group lay on their blankets for 2 hours, moving only to pass around a big bag of potato chips and a bottle of soda. The other group spent most of their time running back and forth from the ocean to a bucket on the sand into which they were dropping various sea creatures they were collecting with nets. The parents spent most of their time in the water or helping their daughters. Those of the blanket group ranged in size from chubby to stout; those of the bucket group were lean or skinny.

The child who does not "burn up" calories in physical activity faces a special problem when he tries to lose weight. He needs very few *calories* but does need the same *nutrients* as a child who never sits down. The foods that supply these nutrients furnish calories as well. To lose weight, the child must eat so little food that he may not be able to obtain all the nutrients he needs.

A program of physical activity is essential to the child who needs to lose weight. It will allow the child to eat more (and obtain his required nutrients) as well as give him some confidence about his body. Since participating in team sports or group activities can be embarassing for the overweight child, he should try some of the recently popular solitary sports such as jogging, bike riding, ice skating, cross-country skiing, or hiking. (Swimming unfortunately requires too much exposure of one's body to be psychologically comfortable for a very overweight child or teenager.) Often the child discovers that his stamina is as good as that of a leaner peer, and although he may not be athletically skillfull, he can run as long, bicycle as far, or climb a mountain as well.

Adult Obesity

Many overweight adults maintain a normal weight throughout childhood, adolescence, and young adulthood. They suddenly find themselves with extra pounds without ever being conscious of overeating, eating compulsively, having food cravings, or even eating fattening foods. Many in this group find it difficult to accept the fact they are overweight because they think of themselves as thin. Often they were thin during childhood and frequently were the subjects of intense efforts to get them to eat more. "What happened?" they ask, "Here I spend the first three decades of my life being told I was too thin and now I need a larger belt."

Most victims of creeping obesity did not notice that changes in their daily routines over the years were affecting their caloric intake and expenditure. Perhaps the most common tendency is for physical activity to decrease while food intake remains the same.

Case 1. A 28-year-old electrician complained that he was rapidly gaining weight and was concerned because his eating habits had not changed over the last 10 years. He did not think he was eating too much because he had eaten considerably more during high school and never gained weight. When asked what he ate, he stated that he lives alone, hates to cook, and takes most of his meals in restaurants. He eats a big breakfast at a local luncheonette (eggs, bacon, toast, butter, hash brown potatoes, coffee with cream). He then gets into his service truck and makes house calls for the next 8 to 9 hours. His only activity is moving from truck to house to truck. Rather then taking time off for lunch, he buys a "submarine" sandwich from a local fast-food shop and eats it in the truck. He frequently spends his evenings drinking beer and eating pizza with friends; otherwise he goes alone to a restaurant and eats the "special" of the day.

He had always been active: football during high school and later on weekend sports with friends and an occasional evening basketball game. Recently his exercise has declined as his friends got married or involved with their own social lives and were not available for a weekend hike or game. It had not occurred to him to join the YMCA or some health club so he would have a place to exercise on a regular basis. Physical activity had once been part of his social life, and he had not yet realized that it should still be part of his daily routine; however, he was unwilling to change his life style so it could be included.

Case 2. In some cases physical inactivity is not the only problem in the generation of excess weight. A 40-year-old businessman complained about his sudden discovery of a second chin and prominent abdomen. "I can't be fat," he exclaimed. "My mother was always forcing me to eat because I was the skinniest kid on the block and the neighbors thought she was starving me."

His daily routine, rather than his eating habits alone, is clearly responsible for his larger suit and belt sizes. He admitted that he rarely moves during the average workday. He commutes to work by train (his wife drives him to and from the station),

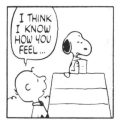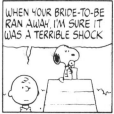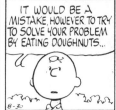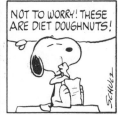

(© 1977 United Feature Syndicate, Inc.)

then takes a subway which stops near his office. He takes an elevator to his office, sits down in a large swivel chair and remains there for the rest of the day. He leaves his office only to take clients to lunch. In the evenings he sits in his office at home and works on the things he cannot finish during the day. He hates exercise and will not consider engaging in any sport. He owns a stationary bike but refuses to ride it because it is boring. He must conduct much of his business over lunch, usually in elaborate restaurants, and he often takes clients to dinner. He never uses these meals as an excuse to overeat; he simply consumes the many items available in a restaurant meal. For example, he has a drink, eats bread and butter while waiting to be served his meal, choses highly caloric salad dressings, adds butter or sour cream to his potato, and pours sauces made with butter and eggs over his fish or meat. He always "cleans his plate" because years of maternal admonitions have affected his adult eating habits. Since restaurants often serve much larger portions than are usually served at home, he might consume 8 ounces of steak or fish, a large potato, several slices of bread, and sometimes a generous portion of dessert.

Meals at home are simpler, but since neither he nor his wife enjoy eating vegetables, they usually fill up on meat or poultry and a salad. The portions of meat are unnecessarily large, since he eats enough protein at lunch to meet his daily requirements. Neither he nor his wife realize that meat can be fattening. Weekends often necessitate dining at the homes of friends, where he eats everything offered lest the hostess be insulted.

Unless this businessman increases his energy expenditure or decreases his caloric intake, he will continue to gain weight and could easily become obese in another few years. There are things he could do to halt the relentless accumulation of pounds. He could get off at a subway stop several blocks away, ride a bicycle to the train station during the warmer months, get a long extension cord on his phone so he could pace around the room while talking, order only salads or appetizers at lunch, or make supper a light meal of soup and a sandwich.

Case 3. The food editor of a newspaper gained 20 pounds the first year of her job. She had to sample recipes, preside over cooking contests, and describe new foods introduced into local supermarkets. She was constantly invited to gourmet lunches and dinners, and was even sent to France and Greece to write about the food. All the diets she tried interfered with her job. Unlike the professional wine or coffee taster, she could not discreetly spit out her samples (hosts and restaurant owners tend to take offence at this). She decided that when she really wanted to reduce, she would simply have to find another type of employment.

Many women's weight problems begin soon after the birth of their first child. They might not lose all the weight gained during pregnancy (this is usually lost within 6 months after giving birth), and often gain more weight with each succeeding child. Pregnancy and motherhood by themselves are not fattening. Here again, changes in a woman's daily routine have conspired to make her consume more calories than she needs. Food is constantly accessible, and opportunities to use up the calories through a regular exercise routine are limited.

Many women who worked up until the time the baby was born have difficulty adjusting to their new lives at home. Long hours of monologues with an attentive but nonverbal baby, "cabin fever" imposed by wintry weather, a sick baby, lack of a car and any place to go, along with 24-hour access to a refrigerator often result in a rapid accumulation of pounds. Caring for colic, teething pains, and endless wet diapers may compel an otherwise self-disciplined and rational mother to seek relief by hitting the cookie jar. As the child grows older, the situation may become even more conducive to weight gain. The cabinets and refrigerator begin to fill up with foods a childless couple rarely include on their shopping list: marshmallow fluff, ice cream on sticks, animal crackers, powdered fruit drink, sugar-coated cereals, cocoa mix, cupcakes, and spaghetti in cans.

Many mothers tend to regard themselves as living disposal units for leftovers and ingest countless extra calories in the form of soggy cereal, bread crusts, and cold spaghetti.

Besides consuming more calories than she needs, the house-bound mother may be utilizing fewer than she suspects. Although she is probably very tired at night, she has not been able to engage in any strenuous form of exercise. She may be picking up, climbing steps, carrying, and walking around constantly, but this routine, though wearing, does not burn up all the calories supplied by melting popsicles and half-eaten apples. However, there are a few simple ways a woman who does not have access to a track or health club or basketball team can exercise to increase her caloric expenditure (without even using a babysitter). For example, she can jump rope for 5 minutes, do exercises for a brief period with or without the help of her child, ride a stationary bike (these can be made cheaply from old bicycles) or take long walks either pushing or pulling a child-occupied vehicle.

The temptation to use the hands to put food into the mouth can be forestalled if the hands or mouth are used for other activities. I took flute lessons when my first child was a baby; knitting or talking on the telephone can also be useful. Getting a goat is probably the best way to dispose of left-overs without guilt, but certain nonfinicky dogs will do as well. (The dog may gain weight but rarely must fit into last year's clothes, so the problem is not serious.)

Lastly, perhaps one of the most effective ways to prevent the accumulation of postpartum pounds is to use a psychological trick borrowed from the behavioral modification method of weight reduction (to be described later). When tedium, loneliness, frustration, or anger propels one to the cabinet or refrigerator, a minute spent writing down the reasons for wanting to eat can often prevent the eating itself. By simply writing, "I am going to finish the banana cake because my children are spilling water on each other, the cat just ate my tunafish casserole, it has been raining for 3 days, and my dryer's broken," one may feel unburdened enough and sufficiently in control to keep that refrigerator door closed a little while longer.

For purposes of description we can put reasons for overeating into two categories, as the case of the housewife–mother illustrates. Overeating may result from fairly straightforward, easily understood *causes* (such as living conditions that present a constant supply of food and little opportunity for exercise) and from less easily understood or dealt with *needs* (such as the need to overeat in response to frustration). The sources of this chronic need to overeat may be psychological or perhaps even biochemical. It is the basic problem to which almost all studies of obesity address themselves and the most difficult type of overeating to control. Moreover, it is generally true that people who want to deal with their own need to overeat usually require some form of outside support and help.

A woman had gained 25 pounds during her first 18 years of marriage. She assumed that her weight gain was related to her forced proximity to a refrigerator during the years she stayed home with her four children. When she continued to gain weight after returning to school, she realized that her reasons for overeating were more conplex than simple access to food. "I could no longer control my eating. I usually started to eat after I fought with the kids or my husband, or when I was trying to contend with the pressures of school and family at the same time. I had tried to diet alone and had failed. I finally decided to sign up for a couse in diet modification when I put on a skirt that had always fit and the button popped off and flew across the room. I know I needed help."

People often find that periods of stress or pressures are alleviated by eating. Styles of eating under stress vary with the individual and the situation, ranging from nervous nibbles to compulsive eating binges. For some, once the stress passes, a decrease in food intake results and the weight gained under stress is lost.

The following cases describe common situations in which people feel the need to overeat.

> *Case 1.* A class of college freshmen and sophomores regarded the week of final exams as one of "unmitigated stress and anxiety." Many endured this period by allowing themselves to eat whatever gave them pleasure. One girl filled her room with cookies she particularly liked; another student ate only nuts and drank soda; and a third ate nothing until late at night when he and his friends would reward themselves for studying by gorging on pizza and beer.

> *Case 2.* A physician told of a situation at his hospital in which the interns and residents often gain weight because they eat excessively at a free midnight supper. Since it is the only relaxation they have, and indeed the only situation free of stress and responsibility, most look forward to the meal and eat copious quantities, regardless of whether they are hungry .

As long as eating alleviates feelings of boredom, anxiety, or anger, it will be used in response to these stresses. An attempt to lose weight during such a period may make the problem seem even more difficult unless new ways of handling the stress are substituted.

> *Case 3.* A young woman gained 30 pounds during her first year of marriage. She and her husband planned to go to medical school, but she had deferred applying for a year and was in graduate school. Her husband had been accepted by a local medical school, and now she was worried that she would not be accepted to one in the same area unless she had excellent grades. "I ate candy bars, doughnuts, and pastries all morning before an exam. After the exam, I was always so worried I hadn't done well I ate ice cream or more candy." She found it impossible to study without a bag of candy by her side. She hated the way she looked and very much wanted to lose weight. However, she admitted that she had no way of handling her anxieties unless she ate (she felt she could not discuss them with her husband because she did not want him to feel guilty about being accepted by the school already); she decided to do nothing about her weight until this aspect of her life was settled.

Sometimes the stress takes years to be resolved. The pattern of overeating adopted in response to stress remains along with the excess weight. It is especially difficult to change that pattern if doing so necessitates thinking about the situation that prompted the overeating. If that situation is simply too painful to be confronted directly, the weight gain will probably be permanent.

> A woman underwent voluntary sterilization after her fourth, accidentally conceived baby was born. Three weeks later her third child suddenly died from an unknown cause, "crib death." This woman, who had been thin all her life, gained 60 pounds during the next year. She may never lose the weight; to do so might necessitate reliving

those tragic days when eating seemed to be the only way of bearing the pain of her child's death and the realization that she could have no more children.

Certain ages may increase an individual's vulnerability to weight gain because of the emotional and social factors which characterize them. For some adolescents and old people, food is one of the few predictable and constant sources of pleasure available.

Excessive weight gain or loss during adolescence is sometimes rooted in psychological events that occurred during childhood. These cases cannot be treated with simple diets or exercise programs. The book *Eating Disorders* (11) furnishes an excellent discussion of the causes for excessive shifts in weight during this period.

Adolescence is a stressful period under the best of circumstances. Pimples that will not go away, a sarcastic teacher, not making the team, not getting invited to a party, and the inevitable friction between parents and siblings are problems many teenagers handle by eating. Food is a source of comfort. Its association with comfort and the relief of pain are believed by many psychologists to be deeply rooted, and although the teenager cannot or will not ask his mother for help or comfort, he can begin to comfort himself the way she used to comfort him—with food.

As the following example illustrates, many adolescents quickly realize that eating provides only temporary relief from their problems.

> A young man in his twenties says that he vividly remembers the first time he responded to stress by overeating. He was about 13 and attended an academically demanding secondary school. One day everything went wrong. He did poorly on a math test, which made him very angry with himself because he liked the subject and usually did well in it. A friend spilled chocolate milk over his Latin assignment, necessitating his redoing it during lunch, an English teacher announced a test on a book he had not finished reading, and during a soccer game after school he made a mistake that lost the game. Tea (actually sandwiches, cookies, and punch) was always served after games and he said he went to it, overcome with a desire to eat. "I gorged myself," he said. "I must have eaten two or three sandwiches, handfuls of cookies and brownies, and I drank several cups of punch. I only stopped when I started to feel sick." He felt terribly guilty at eating so much, but it was the only thing that made him feel better, at least temporarily. He did not really get over the day's events until he went home, vented his anger by fighting with his sister and obtained sympathy by complaining to his mother. "I never ate so compulsively again; I really didn't enjoy it, but every once in a while when I am angry or upset, I find that I still eat much more than I want."

When a teenager's overeating is frequent, attempts to make him lose weight may actually be inadvisable, even though his excess weight can exacerbate the loneliness, low self-esteem, perceptions of rejection by friends and family, and isolation from athletic and social events. If food is his only source of pleasure, a diet will be regarded as yet another type of deprivation. Unless he has a strong desire to lose weight, he may fail to do so, and this failure can decrease his self-esteem even further. Moreover, as an adult who lost 75 pounds in his late twenties said, "I used my obesity as an excuse for my inability to be popular. If I didn't have a date, if I didn't have many friends, if I didn't participate in sports, it was because I was fat."

Weight during adolescence and even young adulthood is *not* predictive of subsequent body weight. Many lean, diet-conscious adults eat their way through adolescence and enter adulthood with 50 to 100 extra pounds. No one, including themselves, would have predicted that they would ever be anything but fat. At some point, however, often when entering a new situation (going away to school, starting a new job, getting married) they decide to lose weight. For many such people, the weight loss is permanent, and eventually (sometimes years later) they stop thinking of themselves as fat; the only people who remember that they had been overweight are relatives who, 20 years after the fact, comment on their loss of weight.

Unfortunately, the events which trigger the transformation of a fat teenager or young adult into a slim individual have never been defined. Each person who goes through such a transformation has his own reasons for doing so, but few have been able to describe how they were able to control their food intake after years of uninhibited eating. These people have not been studied because they cannot be identified. They do not walk through the streets carrying signs proclaiming "I was a fat teenager": and often when they relate their eating history to people who know them only as slim adults, their previous size and gustatory feats are not believed. One hopes that someday their experience and insight can be shared with the present generation of teenagers with weight problems.

An old person's style of eating may change suddenly because of the death of a spouse, sickness, decline in income, or difficulty in food shopping and preparation (see Chapter 8). The diet often becomes very high in carbohydrates (cookies, pastries, bread, cake, crackers) and supplies more calories than are needed. A decrease in physical activity often makes the problem worse. About 50% of older adults in this country are overweight.

It can be very difficult for an old person to lose weight. Merely suggesting a diet or admonishing such an individual to "cut down on calories" is unlikely to help because the eating style of many older people is simply incompatible with caloric restriction. This age group does not routinely fill up on low-calorie bulky foods such as cauliflower, stringbeans, and cucumbers because these foods are difficult to digest. Moreover, the strictly planned meals that characterize many reducing programs are impractical for many older people, especially those who plan eating around socializing: a cup of tea and a doughnut with a friend in the morning, a snack with a neighbor in the afternoon, a group dinner at a fast-food restaurant in the evening. Finally, old people share with teenagers the stresses of a rapidly changing life. Eating a dish of ice cream while watching a late movie on television may be one of the few reliable sources of pleasure to someone trying to get through a long, house-bound weekend.

Older adults who live in housing for the elderly or come together for hot lunches or senior citizen activities can use these opportunities to start and participate in informal weight-reducing groups. Through such groups they can discuss their common problems and share information (such as how to purchase and prepare low-calorie foods). The companionship of such groups might have the secondary effect of diminishing the need to use food as a companion.

The need to overeat is most clearly seen in people who suffer periods of true compulsive eating. Once this type of eating begins, it often does not cease until physical sickness or total exhaustion takes over. Stress may trigger this kind of overeating in certain individuals who learned early in life that eating was an effective distraction from painful and sometimes insoluble emotional problems (12).

> A dramatic description of compulsive overeating in an intensely stressful situation appears in Joyce Carol Oates' novel *Wonderland* (13).
> An adopted son agrees to help his mother escape from the domination of her husband. They go to a hotel, both extremely frightened that they will be discovered and forced to return home. The mother tells the son that she feels faint and shaky; she sends him out for food. He goes to a Chinese restaurant and orders four dinners. When he comes back his mother says, "I was afraid you weren't coming back, Jesse, I'm just so shaky, my nerves are ragged...I feel so faint, I'm dying of hunger." They eat voraciously, and when they finish his mother says that she is still faint from hunger and sends him to get more food. When he returns, he finds that his mother is gone. Apparently, his father has found her and taken her home, leaving behind a note which his son is afraid to read. He squats in the corridor outside the hotel room and eats. "His mouth prickled with each handful of food...his tongue seemed to come alive...Evidently he had been very hungry and had needed this food. There was something desperate in his throat that urged the food down and demanded more. What if he didn't get enough? His stomach was an enormous open hole, a raw hole, a wound. He had to fill it with food. He had to stuff it...His jaw muscles ached from eating...yet he was still hungry. His insides buzzed with hunger...."

Although not all compulsive eaters are overweight (some compensate for periods of insatiable eating with intervals of fasting), the weight gain that results from repeated episodes of this type of overeating is difficult to control. Diet plans, counting calories, and the admonishment to "use a little will power" bear little relationship to the emotional complexities underlying the compulsion to eat. A woman who was successfully losing weight after years of unsuccessful dieting told me that, with the help of a psychotherapist, she finally confronted the situations that made her want to eat compulsively. "I told him that I want to be thin but that I will never stay thin unless I understand why I eat compulsively." Besides recognizing the situations which triggered her eating, she also learned how to replace eating with other types of behavior when she was angry, anxious, or worried.

Factors other than stress also seem to initiate periods of compulsive eating. It is not clear what triggers these "eating spells"; some people seem susceptible to cravings for specific foods, and once they start eating them they may not be able to stop for hours. Eating a doughnut can start a bout of compulsive consumption of sweet foods in a person which ends only when total fatigue or nausea is produced. Some people who are subject to these specific cravings control their eating by never allowing foods that stimulated past eating binges to pass their lips. They are, in fact, similar to recovered alcoholics who never allow themselves one drink because they know they cannot stop with one.

Overeaters Anonymous (discussed in the section on weight loss) is an organization of people who see in themselves a compulsive style of eating. Modeled after Alcoholics Anonymous, the organization supports its members emotionally as well as with diet plans. (Unlike the alcoholic who can give up drinking entirely, the compulsive overeater must continue to eat and thus continuously confronts the temptation to overeat.)

CHARACTERISTICS OF THE OVEREATER

The personalities and eating habits of the overweight have been studied to determine if they are different from those of other people. The premise of these studies is that overweight people may have great difficulty regulating their food intake because their response to food is different from that of normal-weight people. Indeed some psychologists have found that some overweight people tend to eat if the clock indicates it is lunch or dinner time (even if the clock is incorrect), if they are bored, or if the food is particularly tempting or even just accessible. (Working in a bakery or ice cream store may be an "expanding" experience for people who eat warm doughnuts or chocolate chip ice cream if these foods are in front of them.)

The weakness of using this information to solve the problem of overeating among the overweight is that many of the traits described are also found among those whose weight is normal (12). For example, overweight people supposedly eat most of their calories at night. However, many thin people also are night nibblers since they have time and access to a refrigerator or well-stocked pantry. It has also been claimed that the overweight tend to be finicky about the foods they eat; that is, they eat delicious looking and tasting foods even if they are not particularly hungry but will eat little or nothing if the only foods available are tasteless or poorly prepared. However, many people, regardless of their weight, react the same way. If the only foods available for lunch consist of greasy hamburgers, soggy tunafish sandwiches, or rubbery grilled cheese, many eaters skip the meal and "save their calories for something good" (e.g., a fresh chocolate eclair, hot muffin, or gooey pizza).

In his book *American Fried* (14), Calvin Trilling discusses the eating habits of overweight individuals with Dr. Stanley Schacter, a psychologist who has done extensive research in this area. Schacter tells Trillin that "fat Occidentals are much less likely to try chopsticks than thin Occidentals" in Chinese restaurants. Trillin answers:

> "But the fat people behave the way any normal intelligent person would behave, Stanley." He goes on: "I have always thought that anyone who sacrifices stuffing power by using chopsticks in a Chinese restaurant must be demented. I would use a

tablespoon if I thought I could get away with it, but I know the people I tend to share my Chinatown meals with, terrified that I would polish off the twice-fried pork before they had a chance to say 'Pass the bean curd,' would start using tablespoons themselves and sooner or later, we would be off on an escalating instruments race that might end with soup ladles or dory-bailers."

More disturbing is the tendency of some researchers to attribute to the obese person certain personality traits that supposedly explain why he overeats. These traits—low self-esteem, eagerness to please, suppression of anger, lack of assertiveness or confidence, or "jollyness"—are mistakenly thought to precede the uncontrolled overeating which results in obesity. However, many studies have shown that the reverse is true (15). Overweight adolescents and adults are discriminated against, made to feel unworthy, or told that their weight is a sign of weak character or slovenly habits. As a result, many tend to develop a personality to handle society's attitudes toward them, which includes feeling guilty, unworthy, or depressed (15). Hence the "obese personality" is more likely a *response* to the overweight condition than the cause of it. (If people born with curly hair were told that their hair is a sign of laziness, lack of intelligence, or clumsiness, they might also develop feelings of inadequacy and unworthiness.)

People who are overweight are also rumored to have an eating style which differs from those who are thinner. For example, many of them eat quickly and seek situations where they can eat in private, and these traits are thought by some to contribute to their weight problem. However, these eating habits, like personality traits, may be the results rather than the causes of the excess weight. Many overweight people are acutely aware of being watched in restaurants, supermarkets, snack bars, and during social dining. If a thin person and an overweight person sit down at a lunch counter and both order hot fudge sundaes with whipped cream and nuts, the eyes of the other patrons will no doubt be on the heavier person as he receives and begins to eat the ice cream. (In fact, there is a good chance that someone will make some derisive comment about the heavy individual's sundae, such as "Do you see what she's eating? No wonder she's fat!" and totally ignore the thinner person's consumption of the same number of calories.) Under these circumstances, a person would naturally eat quickly, or perhaps even order the sundae in a "take-out" container so it could be eaten in private without the surveillance of other people.

Many people feel compelled to remain overweight although they do not enjoy being that way. Their excess weight becomes an unconscious or even deliberate excuse for failure to achieve their own expectations or those of others. Indeed, since their friends and family often regard this excess weight as a major handicap, they support the belief that failure to attain certain goals is caused by the obesity per se. One often hears family members remark about another who is overweight: "He would get married, have a better job, be accepted into graduate school, or have more friends if only he would lose weight."

The woman mentioned above who had acquired some insight into the reasons for her compulsive eating stated: "I never wanted to get married at 22 and have babies even though this is what my parents expected of me. I gained a lot of weight in college and discovered that my parents stopped worrying about *when* I would get married and began worrying *if*...." She went on to say that she had used her obesity to "excuse my lack of success as an actress, my inability to sustain a close relationship with a man, and my continued financial dependence on my parents."

Of course there is a minority of people who are truly content with their obesity, and the assumption of researchers that all obese people want to lose weight is false.

People who have been overweight since childhood sometimes have feelings about food that are not characteristic of those who became overweight as adults. Some have intense cravings for "fattening" foods that were denied them as children, but they experience painful guilt if they give in to their desires.

> A woman was diagnosed as fat when she was 9 or 10 months old. From that time on her eating was monitored and restricted by her mother. Her siblings and her mother were thin despite their consumption of foods that she was forbidden to eat: ice cream, cookies, potato chips, candies, pies, cakes, muffins, pancakes, and pretzels. Her father was overweight, and when she was older she conspired with him to purchase and hide foods which neither could eat openly in the house. As a result she became overweight. Later as an adult, she was able to lose some weight by participating in various diet organizations; but once she neared her goal she would experience intense cravings for all the foods she had given up during the diet (they were of course the same foods she was denied as a child) and she would then eat them compulsively. Her weight would invariably increase again. She admitted later, when she was taking part in group therapy to help her lose weight, that she never really enjoyed food binges becaue she felt so guilty. Eventually, as a result of therapy, she established a new pattern of eating which included the "forbidden foods." She learned to enjoy them without guilt, and when she found that she could eat them any time she desired she gradually lost her uncontrollable craving for them (16).

WEIGHT LOSS

People gain and keep excess weight when their styles of eating provide more calories then their bodies need. To lose weight, a person must consciously *control* his food intake so he is in caloric deficit; that is, he is taking in fewer calories than he needs.

This control may come easily or with great difficulty, depending on the nature and severity of the weight problem. Some people need only to remind themselves not to eat leftovers while cleaning up after supper (a spoonful of mashed potatoes here, half a frankfurter there) or not to munch absentmindedly on a bowl of nuts after a three-course dinner. Others must change their daily routines to include more exercise and less food. People who chronically overeat because they feel a need to do so may find they are unable to control their eating without some kind of help.

What motivates a person to give up his own eating style, his freedom to eat anything he wishes in any amount, and accept the regulation of a diet? Each successful dieter has his own reasons, and they rarely can be used to inspire another. Guilt after a weekend of overeating is usually not sufficient to sustain dieting for more than 2 or 3 days. Moreover, diets must be started with a fundamental commitment to their authority; otherwise they will be followed only as long as the foods allowed by the diet coincide with those the dieter feels like eating. (The road to dietary failure must be paved with potato chips, ice cream cones, and chocolate chip cookies.)

People succeed in losing weight and maintaining weight loss only when they confront their need for controls on eating. They realize that they must relearn the way they eat and give up their old eating habits, sometimes forever.

The realization that one's eating is out of control is like a window opening for a moment. The person has a strong desire to lose weight, and if he gets encouragement he probably will be successful. If he is dissuaded or does not find a method of weight reduction compatible with his needs, the window shuts, the moment passes, and nothing is done.

> "I had gained about a hundred pounds and I knew I had to lose weight, but I denied both the extent of my weight problem and my ability to handle it." A lean professor was describing the event that began his participation in a long-term diet program. "One morning I came to work thinking that I really wanted to lose weight and admitting to myself that I could not do it without help. Outside my office, I ran into a physician who runs a diet program here. He was in the building because he was giving a seminar that morning. I said to him, 'I want to join your program.' 'Fine,' he replied, 'when do you want to start?' I looked at my calendar and mumbled something about meetings, trips, the end of the semester and pointed to a day several weeks away. 'No, you don't understand,' he said, 'I mean, do you want to see me after the seminar or come to my office this afternoon?' He was right. I never would have started if he had not insisted that I do it immediately. The moment would have passed, and I would have done nothing."

Selecting the Best Method of Undereating

Although making up your mind to diet is obviously the first and most important step in weight reduction, it may be unsuccessful unless a method is chosen that is compatible with your individual desires for food and problems in controlling your eating. Too frequently an overweight person is told to lose some weight by his doctor, relative, or spouse, and then is given a diet plan to follow until the weight is lost. Alternatively, the overweight person might read of a new diet plan in a magazine, hear of a weight loss organization, or see an advertisement for a pill that "melts the fat away" in the back of a magazine and decides that the diet, group, or pill represents the solution to his eating problems. He begins to follow the plan and indeed loses weight. Soon, however, the weight loss decreases, and eventually the plan is discarded and is added to the list of failed diets.

> A member of Overeaters Anonymous told the group that after he had a heart attack his doctor told him he had to lose 40 pounds. "He handed me a list of foods to eat and foods to avoid, and told me to come back when I lost the weight. How could I have lost weight by myself? I used to be an alcoholic, then a chain smoker, and before joining O.A. a compulsive eater. He just didn't understand."

This final section offers a guide to selecting a reducing plan appropriate to your needs. To use it, you must know something about your own eating habits, the reasons for overeating, and whether dieting tends to be more successful when the choice of what and how much to eat is made by someone or something else (e.g., a diet plan or predetermined menu). In addition, some would-be dieters should consider if they would benefit from the availability of an individual or group that offers emotional support, teaches methods for controlling food intake, discusses the reasons responsible for overeating, and finally helps the individual accommodate to a newly emerging thin body.

Counting Calories

A caloric level is set for the dieter so he is eating fewer calories than he needs. Usually the dieter receives a list of foods that will meet his nutritional needs, along with a list of the foods' caloric levels and some suggested menus. Most doctors have such plans, and booklets with this information are available from drugstores, supermarkets, paperback bookstores, and libraries.[2]

Problems with this type of diet include:

1. *Cheating.* It can be difficult for a hungry person to be realistic about the size or weight of food. Several hundred extra calories can be consumed by crediting a food with fewer calories than it actually contains. Hence an apple which rivals a pumpkin in size may be considered "small" by the dieter, or a slab of meat that overhangs the plate and touches the tablecloth may be recorded as a 3-ounce portion.

2. *Losing track of calories.* It is easy to forget to include all the food eaten during a day when tallying up the day's calories. Many people overlook food eaten while standing up, tasted while cooking, or consumed after 11p.m.

3. *Inadequate nutrient intake.* It is possible to eat within a given caloric limit and eat little that is nutritious. A thousand calories worth of potato chips and soda will produce the same weight loss as a thousand calories worth of some more nutritious food. Moreover, if the caloric reduction is severe, the amount of food eaten, however nutritious, may be too small to provide the protein, vitamins, and minerals needed. Unless such a diet is carefully supervised medically and includes appropriate vitamin and mineral supplements, nutritional deficiencies can result.

Calorie-Controlled Meal Plans

A calorie-controlled diet prescribes the types and amounts of foods that may be eaten for each meal. In effect, calories have been precounted for the dieter so he

---

[2]A small booklet, *Calories and Weight* (194-0528-005), is available for $1.00 from the Superintendant of Documents, Government Printing Office, Washington, D.C. 20402.

ingests fewer than he needs if he follows the plan carefully.[3] This type of plan is used by the major weight-reducing organizations: Weight Watchers, Diet Workshop, Diet Watchers, and Overeaters Anonymous. Usually the diets restrict the types and amounts of carbohydrates and fats, and emphasize low-fat cottage cheese, lean meat, and chicken. (The diet suggested by Overeaters Anonymous eliminates foods that are likely to initiate an eating binge and restricts carbohydrates severely since they are associated with overeating.) The fruits and vegetables included provide vitamins, minerals, and bulk with the least calories: mushrooms, stringbeans, tomatoes, kale, spinach, strawberries, citrus fruits, cucumbers, green pepper, etc.)

Recently Weight Watchers and Diet Workshop increased the variety of foods allowed on their plans by setting up an elaborate exchange system. For example, one-half of a bagel can be eaten instead of a slice of bread, and 4 ounces of a low-calorie ice milk in place of a fruit and one serving of milk.

Problems with this type of diet include:

1. *Portion size.* This must be carefully controlled. Everything has to be weighed and measured, even if this necessitates going out to dinner with a scale and measuring cup. Although portion size must also be known on a calorie-counting diet in order for the calorie count to be correct, the eater has more flexibility than on a calorie-controlled diet since he does not have to eat a specified number and types of foods. He can eat a large portion of meat, for example, and, knowing the number of calories it represents, fill up on low-calorie vegetables at a subsequent meal or eliminate a meal entirely to stay within his calorie count. On the calorie-controlled diet plan, all specified foods must be eaten each day. Hence the dieter cannot eliminate one food to compensate for the excess number of calories he may have consumed by eating too large a portion of another.

2. *Rigid adherence to the plan.* The diets are planned so that every item listed for a given meal must be eaten to meet the dieter's daily nutritional needs. People who have erratic eating schedules because of travel, business, school, or vacations may have difficulty obtaining the requisite number of fruit and vegetable servings, for example. Moreover, since the caloric content of the foods is deemphasized, the dieter may not know how to make calorically equivalent substitutions from the foods that are available to him.

Fasting

Fasting is usually carried out in a hospital so the dieter can be medically supervised. The dieter ingests nothing except noncaloric beverages and vitamin and mineral supplements. The method is not commonly used, although it is an effective means of producing rapid weight loss.

---

[3]So long as a diet provides the body with the essential nutrients it needs (vitamins, minerals, protein), the dieter does not suffer from any nutritional deficiency, even though his caloric intake is too low for his body's needs.

Problems with this type of diet include:

1. *Medical Supervision.* Fasting for more than a day or two must be medically supervised.

2. *No new eating habits started.* This type of weight reduction gives the dieter little opportunity to learn a new, controlled eating style to use once he terminates the diet. Often the weight lost by fasting is regained.

Protein-Sparing Diet

With a protein-sparing diet, the dieter goes on a modified fast. He is allowed to eat a small amount of protein each day (2 or 3 ounces of well-cooked lean meat, low-fat cheese, fish, shellfish, or poultry) to replace the protein the body uses up. He must maintain his water intake since the body loses water quickly under these conditions, and he must take vitamin and mineral supplements. A recent book by an osteopathic doctor, Dr. Linn, made this diet popular (17). He advocated using a pure protein preparation rather than foods high in protein.

This type of diet appeals to those who have trouble controlling their food intake even when faced with limited food choices. The protein preparations eliminate all necessity of making decisions about food since the dieter is limited to several tablespoons of the preparation each day. Moreover, people on a protein-sparing diet claim that they stop feeling hungry after a few days. It is thought that high levels of ketones in the circulation may be related to this lack of hunger. [Ketones are compounds produced by the liver from fatty acids (part of the fat molecule) in fat cells. Ketone bodies are produced under normal eating conditions; however, many more are made when no dietary carbohydrate is available.]

Problems with this type of diet include:

1. *Medical supervision.* This diet cannot be followed casually; it must be done under close medical supervision. More than 30 people who were following this diet, eating nothing but a pure protein preparation and vitamin and mineral supplements, have died. Fortunately, deaths from this diet are still rare; however, feeling sick is very common especially for the first few weeks. The dieter can experience a variety of symptoms, including dizziness, nausea, weakness, fatigue, inability to concentrate, muscle weakness, and a decrease in blood pressure. Body levels of certain minerals (e.g., potassium) which the dieter receives through supplements must be checked frequently since individual needs vary. *This is not a "do-it-yourself diet."*

2. *Need for supporting services.* Until this type of diet became fashionable, it was used only by people who needed to lose a considerable amount of weight (50 pounds and up). The success of the diet, as carried out by one of its original proponents, Dr. George Blackburn of the New England Deaconess Hospital, Boston, depends on the supporting services of nutritionists, psychologists, and behavioral modification specialists, who work with the dieter to help him develop a new set of responses and behaviors toward food. The dieter receives supervision also during the transition period from the modified fast to unlimited food choice.

Unless such supportive programs are available, the dieter will probably revert to his old eating pattern once the diet is over. The diet itself does not offer any opportunity to learn new patterns of eating.

3. *Lack of well-balanced eating pattern.* The protein-sparing diet has inspired the creation and sale of diet plans based on protein—*NaturSlim, Nature's Bounty Slim,* and *Figure Food*—which are meant to be substituted for breakfast and lunch. Since these plans do allow a normal third meal to be eaten, they are not really modified fasts. Some of the products contain minerals and vitamins, although the amount and concentration varies among them. Many plans suggest eating nutritionally well-balanced suppers to ensure that the daily nutritional requirements are met. Practically, though, few people are going to eat a third meal which compensates totally for the nutritional deficiencies in the first and second meals (protein powders do not contain all the necessary nutrients). Indeed, according to the *NaturSlim* brochures, "you can sit down to your main meal and enjoy many of the so-called 'forbidden foods.' " These foods very likely do not include bran muffins, lima beans, and kale, and are not selected exclusively for their nutrient content.

Calorie-Controlled Formulated Foods

Cookies or beverages can be purchased that are formulated so a certain number of servings equals 1,000 calories and supplies the adult requirements for eight vitamins and minerals and protein. These foods were very popular a few years ago; Metrecal, Slender, Figurine bars are examples of some products that are still available. They are appealing for some of the same reasons that have made modified protein-sparing diets popular; they decrease the necessity of making any decision about food.

Problems with this diet include:

1. *Lack of bulk.* These "foods" do not provide any bulk and may cause constipation if eaten for prolonged periods of time. (This is probably true of the protein-sparing diets, but with those diets too little food is eaten to make constipation a problem.)

2. *Monotony.* Dieters become bored with the monotony of eating only these foods; the diet seldom works for longer than 2 weeks.

3. *Medical supervision.* Prolonged consumption of these foods alone, without additional vitamin and mineral supplementation, is unwise; these diets, like the protein-sparing diets, require medical supervision.

Unlimited Consumption of Selected Foods

Diets that allow unlimited consumption of certain foods take two forms. One restricts the dieter to one or two foods, sometimes chosen because they supposedly have some special property which, according to the author of the diet plan, "makes the fat melt away." People are told to eat only, for instance, eggs, grapefruit, rice, spaghetti, grapes, or pigs knuckles. Of course these diets lose their appeal before the dieter loses all of his excess weight. They attract people who are bored with conventional diet plans and are looking for some exotic way to lose weight. Unfortunately, few people are able to endure eating only one or two foods.

The other type of diet allows unlimited consumption of protein or of protein plus fat, while restricting or eliminating carbohydrate. The Stillman diet (18), which became popular during the late 1960s, allowed unlimited consumption of protein but restricted fat consumption and severely limited carbohydrate consumption. Atkins published a modification of this plan in 1972 (19). He allowed the dieter to eat all the protein and fat he wished, but eliminated carbohydrate consumption entirely. (Actually neither diet is new; in 1863 William Banting lost 50 pounds by following a similar diet.)

> Banting published *A letter on Corpulence* in 1863 which described his successful weight loss on a diet of meat, fish, and fruit. He was not allowed more than 3 ounces of toast and "rusk" a day, no potatoes, and no milk; but he could have several glasses of sherry. He lost two-and-one-half stone (about 35 pounds) in 9 months (20).

The unlimited quantities of protein allowed on the Stillman diet, and of protein and fat on the Atkins diet, at first remove the feeling of deprivation and self-discipline which surrounds calorie counting and controlled meal plans.

Weight loss is rapid in the early stages because caloric intake falls sharply. Carbohydrates normally supply 40% to 50% of our daily caloric intake. If you can no longer eat bread, pasta, cereal, fruits, vegetables, or any desserts, it becomes difficult to continue eating the same number of calories as before the diet. The diet's apparent initial success is aided by the rapid loss of water that occurs when carbohydrate intake is very low.

Problems with this type of diet include:

1. *Increased cholesterol.* Since these diets are high in cholesterol, they may raise serum cholesterol levels, possibly increasing the risk of heart disease.

2. *Increased urinary ketones.* The Atkins diet stresses elevating ketone bodies in the urine and tells the dieter to test urinary ketone concentration (by using a paper strip which turns a particular color when the concentration is high). However, the high levels of dietary fat may produce an increase in urinary ketone levels that has nothing to do with weight loss.

3. *Medical supervision.* The limited variety of foods allowed by these diets eliminates many sources of vitamins and minerals. Here again, dieting under medical supervision is advisable, and certainly vitamin and mineral supplements should be taken if the diet is followed for more than a week or so. (Iron, riboflavin, vitamin A, and zinc are probably well supplied by the diets; vitamins such as folic acid, pyridoxine, and vitamin C would be lacking, and vitamin D, thiamin, calcium, and potassium may be deficient.)

4. *Side effects.* Few dieters remain on this type of diet long enough to attain their desired weight loss. Many suffer from the side effects of eliminating or reducing

dietary carbohydrate: fatigue, dizziness, inability to concentrate, and loss of strength. Others start to gag as they eat their 13th egg in 5 days: there is a limit to the amount of eggs, fish, meat, chicken, cheese, butter, cream, chicken fat, lard, and pork rinds we can bear to eat.

Diet Modification

Diet modification consists of a program designed to change the individual's eating habits. Based on a form of psychotherapy called behavioral modification, the method combines training in a new style of eating with a low-carbohydrate, calorie-controlled diet. Thus while the individual is losing weight, he is acquiring a new set of eating habits. This approach was introduced in *Slim Chance in a Fat World* by Stuart Davis in 1972 (21) and has been incorporated into the plans of many weight-reduction programs. (Weight Watchers has small group meetings that teach diet modification, and the supervised protein-sparing diet programs like the one described above use it. Some individuals modified the technique further and started their own courses such as Shirley Simon's Learn to be Thin Group in the New England region. A national weight-reduction clinic, The Weight Loss Clinic, uses some aspects of the program.)

Techniques of the program include keeping a careful record of what is eaten every day along with a detailed inventory of where, when, and with whom the eating took place, and, in some programs, the emotions experienced just before eating. (For example, a record might include eating while watching the news on television, at the kitchen table, sitting at the typewriter, cooking dinner, talking with the family, reading and eating apples or ice cream on a bicycle or walking down the street. Emotions might include boredom, frustration when work is not going well, fatigue, impatience, and usually hunger.)

In the next phase of the program. the participant must pay attention to the physical and sensual aspects of food. As he bites, chews, and swallows, he should note whether the food feels slippery, cool, chewy, brittle, grainy, juicy, dry, bulky, smooth, or bumpy. He must concentrate on the food he is eating and stop all other activities. He learns to prolong eating by taking smaller bites, putting the fork down between bites, even getting up from the table and walking around before finishing the meal. (The purpose is to allow the physical feelings of fullness to become apparent.) Other techniques include using small plates so portions look big, always eating in one place (to decrease spontaneous eating), and never eating anything without *first* writing down the food to be eaten. (If you have to write down the planned consumption of a bag of potato chips the temptation is often resisted.) Finally, participants in these programs receive emotional support from other members of their group, the group leader, and their families. Group meetings are often a forum for discussion of the psychological stimuli to overeating; since many of the problems mentioned are common ones, the overeater stops feeling isolated by his eating habits.

Problems with this type of diet include:

1. *Emotional factors.* An effective program must include opportunities to discuss and learn ways of handling the emotional factors that cause overeating. The program fails for people who learn new eating techniques but do not learn how to deal with the emotions which plunged them into overeating in the past.

2. *Timing.* The technique of isolating eating from other activities may be unacceptable to people for whom the social aspects of eating are important.

3. *Inappropriate for impulsive eater.* Since diet modification stresses planning, routine, and orderly eating, it may be inappropriate for the impulsive eater, who is subject to cravings for certain foods. This type of eater need not be overweight because the foods craved are often low in calories and high in nutrients.

Eating Without Guilt

The Psychologist's Eat Anything Book by Pearson and Pearson (22) promotes an alternate diet-modification technique for the impulsive eater. These authors claim that people should become aware of the foods they really want to eat and then eat nothing but those foods. If they eat other foods, they may stop feeling physically hungry but will continue to be psychologically hungry for the foods they really want. If someone has a craving for a piece of fresh bread and butter but does not allow himself to eat it, he may eat excessive quantities of some non-fattening food in a futile attempt to fill up his psychological hunger.

Problems with this type of diet include:

1. *Not suitable for the compulsive overeater.* The authors have not shown that their technique works for the compulsive overeater. Allowing such a person to eat anything might have the same effect as offering a bottle of whiskey to an alcoholic.

2. *Nutrition.* There is no guarantee that the individual's inner hungers will result in food choices that are nutritionally sound. These inner desires may call for a diet of hot fudge sauce, brownies, and chocolate chips.

Comment

Each of these weight reduction methods works for some people. They are effective when their techniques match an individual's particular problem with overeating.

Calorie counting and calorie-controlled meal plans work for people who overeat because of previous inattention to their calorie intake and physical activity. Calorie counting makes inexperienced dieters aware of the caloric content of foods; these people no longer can fool themselves into thinking that a salad sinking under the weight of its dressing has no calories, or that a chiffon pie or chocolate mousse is not fattening because it is "full of air." A person who has gained expertise in calorie counting has the advantage of being able to eat a wide variety of foods. He can eat that chiffon pie because he has eliminated something with an equal number of calories from another meal. (This is not a recommendation for eating desserts!)

Some people prefer to give the responsibility of choosing their foods to someone else. These dieters succeed by joining a weight-reducing organization that provides a controlled meal plan and weekly weight check; by convincing someone close to them to select, weigh and measure their food; or by following a single-food diet plan which eliminates all need to make food choices. (The protein-sparing diets appeal to such people).

> Enjoyment of food is an important part of some people's lives. A woman who loves to eat and cook spends most of her spare time either giving or going to dinner parties. About twice a year she discovers that she has gained 15 or so pounds and temporarily hands control of her eating to Weight Watchers. She says, "I have to have someone controlling what I eat and watching my weight. If I know I will be weighed every Monday, I can stay on their diet over the weekend. I cannot follow their plan without the support of the meetings and the woman who runs them."

Profit-making weight reduction clinics are appearing now in major cities and their suburbs. These clinics promise immediate and persistent weight loss, and are probably able to live up to these promises as the method they use exerts tight control over what the dieter eats. The dieter is given little choice over the foods he can select; the diet is a 500-calorie, low-carbohydrate meal plan, and the nutrient deficiencies on such a limited diet are compensated with daily vitamin and mineral supplements. The dieter is weighed each weekday and must come in for the weighing and to obtain his vitamin-mineral supplement for the following day. (He is never weighed on Sundays! He gets two supplements on Saturday for use on Sunday and Monday.) The almost daily weight loss appears to reinforce the dieter's desire to stay on the diet for yet another day; however, two other factors also influence his continued dieting. The first is that the plan is expensive and prepaid; therefore dropping out means a loss of money. The second is that the staff members call a client who does not show up for the daily weigh-in and first remind and then "nag" him to come in. They are very persistent, and the only way to escape the relentless phone calls is to drop out of the plan.

Diet-modification groups or groups such as Overeaters Anonymous, which combine dieting with emotional support and techniques for understanding and modifying eating behavior, are very effective for people whose weight problem results from an inner need to overeat. A dieter's family can provide excellent support, encouraging him to keep up the diet, even when he faces some culinary temptation.

> A woman who joined the diet-modification class said that after she had lost some weight her children were so pleased they helped her stay on the diet. When she felt an irresistible desire for ice cream, they would hear her open the freezer door and come into the kitchen. As she was taking out the ice cream they would tell her, "Mom, don't eat that, you look so great now, it would be awful if you started to gain weight again." This was enough to keep her from eating it.

Weight-reducing groups are another source of emotional support. In some, members are weighed at weekly meetings and applauded for weight loss or offered sympathy if none has occurred. The groups allow members to discuss mutual problems: what to eat at the home of a friend if no food is served that is on the diet plan, how to refuse dessert without offending the hostess, or how to prevent nibbling when the dieter is preparing dinner (one club suggests wearing a surgical mask).

Weight-reducing groups can also provide a forum for discussing the special problems faced by those who are losing large amounts of weight and gaining a new body shape and sometimes a new personality.

> Women often say they are shy about seeing their husbands and friends after just having had a permanent. Indeed they have trouble recognizing themselves in the mirror with their suddenly acquired curly hair. When people acquire a totally new body from prolonged dieting, they experience the same strangeness except it lasts longer and is more intense.

Overeaters Anonymous is a nonprofit organization modeled after Alcoholics Anonymous, with chapters in most cities. Members believe that they are never "cured" of their desire to eat compulsively no matter how long their weight has been stable. They regard each day as a new challenge and a new opportunity to control their eating; they believe the challenge can be met with the support of the other members and God. Because people share with each other stories of their excessive and sometimes bizarre eating, no one feels peculiar because of the way he eats. As one member said, "If someone stands up and says that he ate a dozen doughnuts, someone else will say, 'Is that all?' and tell how he ate a dozen doughnuts and a pie; and then someone else will say he has eaten a dozen doughnuts, a pie, and a quart of ice cream."

The organization suggests a diet, and each new member is urged to find a sponsor (another member) with whom he checks the foods he plans to eat each day. He must receive approval for his choice of foods and cannot make changes without first consulting a member. He is also encouraged to seek emotional support from members with whom he can discuss the reasons for his overeating. The meetings are run by volunteers; there are no dues, although a small voluntary contribution is requested at each meeting. In many areas, meetings are held during the day and evening, every day of the week. Often a new member is sustained through the early months of dieting by attending meetings every night. People continue to attend meetings years after they have achieved a satisfactory weight. One woman who had lost weight 9 years earlier said that she still needed the support of the group.

An individual who diets over a long period especially needs emotional support, even if his reasons for overeating are fairly easy for him to deal with.

> The dieter is constantly and deliberately denying himself one of the primary components of life, food. Although he may not be physically hungry, he may be

psychologically hungry since he can no longer use food as a source of comfort or pleasure. The man who successfully lost a hundred pounds over a year said, "It is impossible to sustain long-term dieting without the continuous love and encouragement of someone else. Dieting is very lonely. Since the novelty of losing weight stops after the first few months, and you know you still have months to go before your goal is reached, you must develop your own discipline to continue fighting the temptation to give up. Unless someone is right here giving you support and reason to go on, it is very easy to quit."

A man at Overeaters Anonymous who had lost 75 pounds and had another 50 to go said, "As the fat goes away, all sorts of problems emerge. For example, I had been fat all my life and used it to avoid social interaction with girls. Now I am just learning how to ask a girl out on a date and how to act, things you usually learn as a teenager. The only people I can ask for advice are other members who have gone through the same experience. Anyone else would laugh at me."

An individual who must stay on a diet for a year or more should try to find a program with a well-developed support system. He needs more than a reducing plan; he needs to learn behavioral modification to help him maintain his weight loss after the diet is completed; he needs also to have a psychologist available with whom he can discuss the complex emotional reasons for his overeating, his frustration and anger over the chronic self-denial of the diet, and his worries about handling his new image as a thin person. The most successful of such plans also include opportunities for the dieters to meet with each other so their mutual successes or problems can be shared. Some programs include the services of a nutritionist who instructs the participants in methods of choosing foods to meet their nutrient needs when their caloric intake is limited.

The people closest to a long-term dieter may also have difficulty adjusting; they may actually try to discourage continuation of the diet. The reasons vary. A spouse may feel threatened when the person he married begins to take on an entirely different shape. The increasing attractiveness of the partner (and often increasing assertiveness) may change the entire relationship.

"I no longer swallow my anger by eating compulsively," said a woman who had already lost almost 70 pounds. "Now I get angry and my husband and friends don't know how to relate to me. My husband said he liked me better before I lost my weight."

A special relationship can develop between an overweight parent and child if they share in the guilt of secretly eating forbidden foods. Should one and not the other start to lose weight, the other may feel angry and isolated.

A young woman said that she was unable to lose weight until she left home. Both she and her father were overweight and had worked out a system for buying snack foods for each other and hiding them in the house. When she was about 15 she decided to lose weight and joined a local diet club. "I never reached the weight I wanted to be," she said. "When I was about 15 pounds from my goal, my father told me that I looked wonderful and should stop the diet. We were at the kitchen table. He then handed me a piece of cake and said 'Eat it.' I knew if I didn't he would be very angry at me and I couldn't stand that. I went off the diet and eventually gained back all the weight I had lost."

No one should be pushed, threatened, cajoled, or bribed onto a diet. A person who has been considerably overweight for many years does not undertake a long-term diet casually. In addition to committing himself to months of food deprivation and denying his former eating habits, he exposes himself to the risk of failure. (Losing 75 to 100 pounds is *not* the same as dieting for a few days or weeks.) When a person starts to diet, he has a particular goal in mind. Should he stop before he reaches it, he will feel that he has failed regardless of how much weight he loses. Many people who are chronically overweight have a rather low regard for themselves, and failure does not help anyone's self-esteem or future chances of success.

Dieting and maintaining weight loss do not rank among the world's greatest pleasures. Each individual must decide for himself if he is willing to undertake this rewarding but painful process.

In *American Fried* (14), Calvin Trillin asks Fats Goldberg, a reformed overeater who went from 320 to 160 pounds, if losing and keeping off the weight is worth the effort.

> "Well, I figure that in my first 25 years, I ate enough for four normal lifetimes," Fats said. "So, I get along. But there is a lot of pain involved. A lot of pain. I can't stress that enough."

Finally, there are those who are content with their style of eating and their shape. To them, an excerpt from the poem *Teddy Bear* by A. A. Milne (23) is offered:

> A bear, however hard he tries,
> Grows tubby without exercise
> Our Teddy Bear is short and fat,
> Which is not to be wondered at,
> But do you think it worries him
> To know that he is far from slim?
> No, just the other way about—
> He's *proud* of being short and stout.

REFERENCES

1. Garn, S.M., and Clark, D.C. (1976): Family line origins of obesity. In: *Second Wyeth Nutrition Symposium,* edited by L.A. Barnes, pp.3–13. Wyeth Laboratories, Philadelphia.
2. Garn, S.M., Clark, D.C. and Ullman, B. (1975): Does obesity have a genetic basis in man? *Ecol. Food Nutr.,* 4:57.
3. Garn, S., Bailey, S., and Higgins, I. (1976): Fatness similarities in adopted pairs. *Am. J. Clin. Nutr.,* 29:1067.
4. Mayer, J. (1974): *Human Nutrition.* Charles C. Thomas, Springfield, Ill.
5. Sheldon, W.H. (1940): *Varieties of Human Physique.* Harper, New York.
6. Knittle, J., and Hirsch, J. (1968): Effect of early nutrition on the development of rat epididymal fat pads. *J. Clin. Invest.,* 47:2091.
7. Editorial (1974): Infant and adult obesity. *Lancet,* Jan. 5:17.
8. Charney, E.H.G., McBridge, M., Lyon, B., and Pratt, R. (1976): Childhood antecedents of adult obesity. *N. Engl. J. Med.,* 295:6.
9. Wilkinson, P., Pearlson, J., Parkin, J., Philips, P., and Sykes, P. (1977): Obesity in childhood: A community study in Newcastle-upon-Tyne. *Lancet,* 12:350.

10. Poskitt, E., and Cole, T. (1977): Do fat babies stay fat? *Br. Med. J.,* 1:7.
11. Bruch, H. (1973): *Eating Disorders.* Basic Books, New York.
12. Meyer, J.D. (1976): Psychopathology and eating disorders. In: *Appetite and Food Intake,* edited by T. Silverstone. Abakon Verlags-gesellschaft, Berlin.
13. Oates, J. (1971): *Wonderland.* Fawcett, Greenwich, Conn.
14. Trillin, C. (1974): *American Fried.* Doubleday, New York.
15. Bruch, H. (1979): Obesity. In: *Nutrition and the Brain,* Vol. IV, edited by R. Wurtman and J. Wurtman *(in press).*
16. Kales, E., therapist of weight-reducing group called Feeding Ourselves: personal communication.
17. Linn, R. (1977): *The Last Chance Diet.* Bantam, New York.
18. Stillman, I.M., and Baker, S.S. (1967): *The Doctor's Quick Weight Loss Diet.* Prentice Hall, Englewood Cliffs, New Jersey.
19. Atkins, R.C. (1972): *Dr. Atkins's Diet Revolution.* McKay, New York.
20. Drummond, J.C., and Wilbraham, A. (1939): *The Englishman's Food.* Jonathan Cape, London.
21. Stuart, R.B., and Davis, B. (1972): *Slim Chance in a Fat World: Behavioral Control of Obesity.* Research Press, Champaign, Ill.
22. Pearson, L., and Pearson, L. (1973): *The Psychologist's Eat Anything Book.* Popular Library, New York.
23. Milne, A.A. (1924): Teddy Bear. In: *When We Were Very Young.* Dutton, New York.

5 EATING FOR TWO:
Nutrition During Pregnancy

The objectives of the dietary recommendations for pregnancy are:

1. To furnish an optimal supply of nutrients for the growth of the fetus as well as the storage of certain of these nutrients for use after birth.

2. To provide nutritional support for the growth of maternal tissue.

3. To prevent depletion of the maternal nutrient reserves.

HISTORY

Today the medical profession generally accepts the fact that a nutritionally inadequate diet during pregnancy can affect the pregnancy's outcome, either by preventing optimal development of the fetus or by causing nutrient deficiencies in the mother. A well-defined prenatal diet and the use of dietary supplements are now standard aspects of prenatal care. Concern about the dietary implications of pregnancy is a new concept, however. As recently as the beginning of this century, the diets of pregnant women were either ignored, treated casually, or modified in such a way as to be potentially harmful to both mother and fetus (1).

Early in this century a Russian doctor proposed feeding women a diet containing adequate protein but limited amounts of carbohydrate and fluid. Physicians in the United States followed his dietary recommendations well into the 1920s (1). The diet may have contained sufficient protein, but the restriction in carbohydrate (including fruits, vegetables, and grains) must have curtailed the intake of vitamins and minerals. Total caloric intake was also restricted by this diet, and this restriction became acceptable medical procedure for decades because the baby at birth would be normal in length but very thin (i.e., deficient in fat tissue). The birth of such an infant was easier than delivering a baby with normal fat stores, especially if the woman had a small or malformed pelvis (sometimes the result of childhood rickets). Underfeeding the mother was considered the only dependable method of retarding the growth of the fetus; the alternative—delivering a normal-size child—could necessitate a cesarean section, which at that time was a risky procedure.

The weight gain of pregnant women was also limited for another reason: to prevent the complication known as toxemia. Toxemia is a complex of symptoms that includes edema (swelling) of the hands and face, protein in the urine, and in some cases an acute elevation of blood pressure (2). Whether limiting the amount of weight gained during pregnancy can prevent the symptoms of toxemia has been disputed for years; however, women have long been admonished to keep their weight gains within rather strict limits (18 to 20 pounds) to prevent its occurrence.

The current consensus is that "there is no evidence that women with large total weight gain due to excessive accumulation of fat are more likely to develop toxemia than women with lesser accumulation" (2).

A severe reduction in caloric intake is often accompanied by a reduction in the intake of nutrients, because the amount and variety of foods that can be consumed on such a diet are small. Women who were forced to adhere to an extremely restrictive diet to prevent what is considered today to be a normal weight gain during pregnancy (24 to 25 pounds) may not have been able to eat the vitamins, minerals, and protein considered necessary by today's standards.

However, the nutritional inadequacy of the woman's diet was not considered a problem during the early part of the century. Many physicians believed that the fetus functioned as a parasite—i.e., it obtained all the nutrients it required from the mother (as a tapeworm might from its host) regardless of what she ate. This belief has been refuted by much research that documents the effects of protein, vitamin, and mineral deficiencies on the nutritional status of the child (2–5). In addition, insufficient intake of calories seems to be related to the birth of babies with weights of 5 pounds or less; these infants are called "small-weight-for-date" babies, and their health and even survival at birth are precarious.

Today women who eat calorically insufficient diets are given food supplements to increase the weights of their babies at birth. This practice directly contradicts earlier theories of prenatal care, which, as we have seen, considered the birth of a 5-pound or smaller baby as evidence that the dietary objectives had succeeded.

Today no one would dispute the contention of many grandmothers that the pregnant woman is indeed "eating for two" (although, as one obstetrician said, not for two adults). What the pregnant woman should eat has now been well established; long lists of nutrient requirements are available (Table 1), and the lists are continually revised as laboratory and clinical studies define more precisely the quantity and type of nutrients needed by the woman and her fetus.

NUTRIENTS AND THE STAGES OF PREGNANCY

Specific changes occur in the fetus and mother over the 9-month gestation, and these changes are the basis on which nutrient requirements for pregnancy are established. Pregnancy is divided into three periods (trimesters), and specific maternal and fetal developments occur during each period. No one would confuse an 8-month pregnant woman with one only 2 months pregnant; visible differences exist between the two because of events that happen during one trimester and not the other. More subtle changes also occur during each period, although there is no sharp line dividing one trimester from the next.

> A woman who suffered acutely from morning sickness fully expected (at least hoped) that on the *first* morning of the second trimester the nausea would be gone. To her disappointment, it was not.

Nevertheless, the timing of various maternal and fetal events during each

TABLE 1. *Recommended Daily Dietary Allowances*[a]

Nutrient	Pregnancy requirement	Increase over nonpregnancy requirement
Energy	2,400 cal	300 cal
Protein	76 g	30 g
Vitamin A[b]	1,000 RE or	200 RE or
	5,000 IU	1,000 IU
Vitamin D_2	400 IU	No change
Vitamin E	15 IU	3 IU
Ascorbic acid	85 mg	15 mg
Folacin (folic acid)	800 mg	400 mg
Niacin		
Age 19–22 years	16 mg	2 mg
Age 23–50 years	15 mg	2 mg
Riboflavin		
Age 19–22 years	1.7 mg	0.3 mg
Age 23–50 years	1.5 mg	0.3 mg
Thiamin	1.3 mg	0.3 mg
Vitamin B_6	2.5 mg	0.5 mg
Vitamin B_{12}	4 mg	1 mg
Calcium	1,200 mg	400 mg
Phosphorus	1,200 mg	400 mg
Iodine	125 μg	25 μg
Iron	36 mg	18 mg
Magnesium	450 mg	150 mg
Zinc	20 mg	5 mg

[a]These recommendations are based on a woman weighing 128 pounds who is 5 feet 2 inches tall and is between the ages of 19 and 50.

[b]Vitamin A requirements are expressed in two ways: as RE (retinol equivalents) and as IU (international units).

trimester has been well defined. Toward the end of the first trimester, the placenta and amniotic fluid[1] are formed, and by the end of the second month the major organ systems of the fetus have started to develop. During the second trimester (4 to 7 months), the mother's body undergoes noticeable physiologic (functional) changes: increases occur in the volume of her blood and in breast and uterine tissues. In addition, fat is being stored in maternal fat depots, which developed sometime during our evolution to serve an important function after birth. The stored fat provides enough energy to meet the caloric cost of nursing a baby for about 3 months. Hence a woman's ability to lactate (produce milk) is not totally dependent on the number of calories she eats, at least for the first few months after her baby's birth. Although the mother who bottle-feeds her infant may view these fat reservoirs with the same enthusiasm she reserves for her maternity clothes, these deposits do aid the breast-feeding mother who may find herself still trying to finish her breakfast at dinner time.

---

[1]The placenta is the tissue that transfers nutrients and oxygen from the mother to the fetus. It can weigh 350 to 1,000 grams at birth. The amniotic fluid supports the fetus and cushions it against mechanical injury.

Some of the specific nutrient requirements of pregnancy (e.g., the increased needs for calories and iron) are based partially on changes in the mother's body. These requirements and others are also related to the ongoing process of growth and development in the fetus. Much of the actual development of the fetus is completed before many women even realize they are pregnant. As mentioned earlier, after 8 weeks the organs and skeleton have started to form. Although no conclusive evidence indicates that a lack of certain nutrients very early in pregnancy can produce malformations of the fetus, common sense dictates that a diet of only black coffee and yogurt be avoided when pregnancy is suspected.

In general, most of the nutrient requirements are based on the rapid rate of fetal growth that starts during the third month and continues until birth. At the beginning of the second trimester, a fetus may weigh 7 ounces and be 6 inches long. By birth, he will have almost quadrupled his length and will weigh, on the average, slightly more than 7 pounds. The baby's body will contain enough iron to support new red blood cell formation for 3 months or more, a 24-hour supply of stored glucose,[2] and sufficient body fat to insulate his body from heat loss at birth. (When a baby is born, he is transported from a maternal temperature of approximately 98.6°F to a room temperature of about 75°F.) Nutrients for these developments come from the mother—from her internal stores as well as her diet. What then should her diet contain to support this rapidly growing life within her?

NUTRIENT REQUIREMENTS OF PREGNANCY

The nutritional requirements of pregnancy fall into three categories: calories, protein, and vitamins and minerals. Carbohydrates (sugars and starches) and fats are not required in any specific amount during pregnancy (or, for that matter, during normal conditions). Carbohydrates are usually included in the pregnant woman's diet because they are a source of energy and of vitamins and minerals.[3] The fetus and its mother also need fat because of a particular fatty acid (linoleic acid[4]), which is contained in the structure of simple fats. Moreover, a certain class of vitamins, called fat-soluble vitamins (A, D, K, and E), are also associated with the fat component of food. However, since fat is rarely lacking in the diet (fat pills are noticeably absent from the multitude of dietary supplements sold in drugstores), the pregnant woman need not be concerned with obtaining sufficient fat in her diet. Table 1 lists the nutrient requirements of the pregnant woman.

---

[2]Glucose is stored in the liver in the form of glycogen.

[3]Enriched flour products (e.g., breads, pasta, and fortified cereals) are carbohydrates that provide many of the B-complex vitamins. In addition, fruits and vegetables, which are low-carbohydrate foods, are good sources of a variety of vitamins and minerals.

[4]Linoleic acid cannot be made by the body. In addition to its role in the structure of some fats (triglycerides), it is needed for the formation of another fatty acid (arachidonic acid), which is involved in the synthesis of a group of chemicals called prostaglandins.

Calories

Caloric intake should increase by 300 calories a day. The pregnant woman needs more calories because placental and fetal growth require energy, and, in addition, the woman is continuously carrying around several extra pounds of fetal, placental, and other tissues associated with pregnancy. This recommended caloric increase assumes that the woman will continue a level of activity during pregnancy that is comparable to her activity before she became pregnant. Obviously, if she chooses to spend the 9 months in bed, her caloric needs may actually decrease. Conversely, should her pregnancy coincide with a 4-month hike through the Rockies, then her caloric intake must be adjusted upward.

When in doubt about total daily caloric intake, a rule of thumb is the following: The number of calories per day should not fall below 36 calories per kilogram of body weight (or 16 calories per pound). If the caloric intake drops below that level, then the body will use the protein supplied in the diet for its energy needs rather than its protein needs.

The food equivalent of an extra 300 calories a day is disappointingly small. Visions of three banana splits should vanish when you consider that a piece of cherry pie contains 303 calories and one 3-ounce serving of roast pork contains 310. Nevertheless, the increase in calories may make it somewhat easier for the pregnant woman to eat the nutrients she needs since the amount or variety of foods she can choose increases slightly.

Weight reduction during pregnancy is usually not recommended by obstetricians (2) primarily because a reduction in caloric intake is usually accompanied by a reduction in nutrient intake (the less you eat, even of broccoli and cottage cheese, the fewer vitamins, minerals, and protein you obtain). Doctors feel that supplying sufficient nutrients to both fetus and mother is more important than producing a weight loss in the mother, although few discourage a prospective mother from cutting out desserts or potato chips. In general, strenuous dieting is recommended only before or after pregnancy. Finally, dieting during pregnancy is difficult psychologically; it is very hard to be convinced that a diet is successful when the only visible loss is one's figure.

The standard weight gain during pregnancy is about 24 pounds, but the weight a normal individual can gain ranges from 20 to 30 pounds, and occasionally, with monitoring by one's obstetrician, it can be even more. Sometimes an underweight woman is encouraged to gain additional weight during pregnancy so her weight after birth will be closer to normal. The first trimester produces very little weight gain—usually a total of 1.5 to 3 pounds. During the second and third trimesters, weight gain is more rapid owing to the ever-increasing size of the fetus and maternal tissue (e.g., the placenta); the weight gain averages about 0.8 pound per week, or 1 pound every 9 days.

A 25-pound gain in weight is not considered excessive because it approximates the combined weights of all the products of gestation: fetus, placenta, increased blood volume, maternal fat stores, and enlarged breast tissue. However, as recently as 10 or 15 years ago, women were told not to gain more than 20 pounds in order to prevent the development of toxemia. As a result, women who gained more than 20 pounds by the beginning of their ninth month often resorted to various subterfuges to disguise their weight gain: they wore their lightest clothes to the doctor's office (bathing suits in February) or fasted the day before. The present flexibility among obstetricians regarding their patients' weight gain reflects the findings of current studies—that no relationship exists between the incidence of toxemia and a weight gain of up to 30 pounds (4).

Protein

Thirty additional grams of protein is needed each day during pregnancy, bringing the total protein requirement to 76 grams. Although this may seem like a lot, eating this much protein is usually not difficult for the typical American. Table 2 lists the protein content of some commonly eaten foods, and by quickly adding up the number of grams you can see how easy it is to eat over 76 grams in a day. The pregnant woman should also include three or four glasses of milk in her daily diet, and, at 9 grams of protein for an eight-ounce glass of milk, she may easily end up consuming around 100 grams of protein a day.

The foods listed in Table 2 represent *animal protein,* which is the usual form of protein recommended in lists of nutrient requirements. Animal protein refers not only to food from four-footed animals chewing grass; it also includes eggs, milk, dairy products, fish, and forms of meat other than beef. (Women in Botswana eat porcupine.) Protein is also found in nonanimal foods, e.g., wheat and other cereal grains, nuts, legumes (kidney beans), seeds (pumpkin, sesame, sunflower), and to a small extent fruits and vegetables. Protein from nonanimal sources is called *vegetable protein.*

The body is not able to use vegetable protein as efficiently as animal protein because of differences in essential amino acid content. Proteins are composed of two types of amino acids: essential and nonessential. Eating supplies our bodies with essential amino acids; the nonessential amino acids can be made by the body and are therefore "nonessential" to the diet. Animal proteins are the better source of the nine essential amino acids because they contain these compounds in the

TABLE 2. *Protein content of some foods*

Food	Protein (grams)
Tunafish (3 oz)	24
Cottage cheese (1 cup)	33
Hamburger (3 oz)	21
Egg	7
Pizza (2 slices)	14
Ham (3 oz)	18
Chicken salad (½ cup)	25

proportions needed by the body for making its own protein.[5] Vegetable protein, on the other hand, may contain an insufficient amount of one, or sometimes two, of the essential amino acids. A protein that lacks sufficient amounts of one or more essential amino acids is often called an *incomplete protein;* conversely, a *complete protein* is one that contains essential amino acids in the amounts appropriate for use by the body. Since proteins from different types of nonanimal food (e.g., seeds or grains) are not deficient in the same essential amino acids, you can obtain all the required essential amino acids by combining vegetable proteins with different amino acid deficiencies. Eating complementary proteins (i.e., those proteins whose combined amino acid composition equals that of animal protein) is something that knowledgeable vegetarians have been doing for years and which many cultures have practiced, perhaps unwittingly, for centuries. Beans and rice, sesame seed paste and wheat, corn meal and beans are three examples of complementary proteins that are currently eaten together in various parts of the world and different ethnic enclaves in the United States.[6]

Because of the higher cost of animal protein, a pregnant woman on a limited income may not be able to buy and eat the recommended quantity of 76 grams per day. Theoretically, she should be able to obtain the protein she needs from the correct combination of foods. However, planning meals around complementary protein foods is not automatic, especially for those whose ethnic background does not include such dishes as tacos with refried beans or tahini (sesame seed paste) with Syrian bread. A certain amount of nutritional expertise, motivation, and time are required to prepare such foods properly (it takes longer to cook rice and beans than to open a can of spaghetti); in addition, these foods must appeal to the eater. The mother who is poor may therefore go through pregnancy eating insufficient amounts of complete protein and, depending on the degree of inadequacy, increase the risk of retarded growth in her developing baby. As mentioned earlier, babies weighing less than 5 pounds at birth, after a full 9-month pregnancy, are known as small-weight-for-date babies. The cause for the smaller than normal size is often related to either protein or protein-calorie deficiencies during pregnancy: Mothers who had previously given birth to such small-for-date babies were able to produce normal-size babies during subsequent pregnancies when their diets were supplemented with foods containing recommended amounts of complete protein (5).

Because of this risk to fetal health when pregnant women cannot obtain enough animal protein, the government has developed and funded a new program to provide high-quality protein foods to women who cannot afford to buy them. This

---

[5]New proteins are synthesized by the body from available essential and nonessential amino acids. If the supply of certain essential amino acids is limited, protein synthesis stops when they are used up, even if the others are still available. This process is similar to stringing a necklace from red, blue, and yellow beads and stopping when the yellow ones are all gone.

[6]Francis Moore Lappe's *Diet for a Small Planet* (Ballantine Books, New York, 1971) is an excellent reference for information about complementary proteins and how to use them in foods that taste good.

program, known as WIC,[7] supplies women with coupons redeemable for animal protein foods such as milk, eggs, cheese, and meat.

Vitamins and Minerals

Predictably, the rapid growth of the fetus and the development of maternal tissues result in a considerable increase in vitamin and mineral requirements during pregnancy. Many of these vitamins and minerals are stored in the mother's body in limited quantities (the B vitamins and vitamin C, for example) and must be replaced constantly by nutrients in the daily diet. Even those nutrients that are stored in ample amounts (e.g., calcium) must eventually be replaced by dietary sources. A woman who goes through pregnancy eating only negligible amounts of calcium is like a person who continually writes checks without depositing any money; at some point a time of reckoning occurs. This point may come when the woman is in her sixties and breaks a hip or notices that she is shrinking!

Eating (vitamins and minerals) for two does not necessitate eating twice as much. As Table 1 shows, many of the requirements increase only slightly above nonpregnant levels and can be reached without totally disrupting the mother's previous eating style (unless, of course, the prepregnant diet was strong on potato chips and weak on carrots and dark green leafy vegetables).

However, not all of the increased nutrient requirements are satisfied easily. A pregnant woman needs three nutrients—calcium, folic acid, and iron—in amounts significantly greater than are needed before pregnancy, and to obtain them she may have to select deliberately those foods that are good sources of these nutrients. Physicians often recommend supplements (vitamins and mineral pills) to avoid the uncertainty of whether their patients will obtain their requirements from daily food choices. Very few women tabulate the vitamin and mineral content of their day's food intake to determine if they ate sufficient amounts of iron, and even fewer cook themselves some liver at 11 p.m. if they find they did not eat enough iron during the day.

Calcium

As everyone learns in second grade, calcium is an essential mineral for the formation and maintenance of the skeletal structure and the development of the teeth. In addition (and not mentioned in second grade), calcium has indispensable roles in the function of the nervous system, contraction of muscles, coagulation of blood, and beating of the heart muscle.

The fetus needs large amounts of calcium as it develops these functions and structures, and as gestation progresses the amount the fetus takes from its mother increases. Much of the calcium that is present in a newborn baby—approximately

---

[7]WIC stands for Special Supplemental Food Program for Women, Infants, and Children, and is funded by the U.S. Department of Agriculture.

TABLE 3. *Calcium content of some foods*

Food	Calcium (grams)
Sardines (3 oz)	0.3
Enriched macaroni and cheese (1 cup)	0.3
Pizza (⅛ of a 14-inch one)	0.1 (who eats only one piece?)
Homemade spaghetti (1 cup)	0.12
Canned tomato soup, made with milk (1 cup)	0.17
Clam chowder, made with milk (1 cup)	0.24
Oyster stew, made with milk (1 cup)	0.3
Broccoli (1 stalk)	0.15
Spinach (1 cup)	0.2
Canned salmon (2/5 cup)	0.25
Rice pudding with raisins (¾ cup)	0.14
Chocolate pudding (¾ cup)	0.14
Custard pie (1/6 of 9-inch one)	0.14
Vanilla ice cream (¼ qt)	0.2
Alligator meat (3.5 oz)	1.23 (one alligator should provide enough calcium for an entire pregnancy!)

25 to 28 grams (about 1 ounce)—is deposited during the last trimester. A large daily intake of calcium must thus be maintained throughout pregnancy, and the ninth month especially is no time for the mother-to-be to stop drinking milk.

In the nonpregnant individual about two-thirds of the calcium eaten never makes the critical passage across the wall of the intestine to enter the bloodstream (so that it will be delivered to the cells). Instead, much of the ingested calcium is excreted with other intestinal wastes. During pregnancy, however, the absorption of calcium into the bloodstream is more efficient, ensuring the availability of this mineral for both fetal and maternal needs (assuming, of course, that the recommended amount of calcium is eaten). Some of this calcium is stored within the mother's body to be used after birth when nursing her baby.

As Table 1 shows, the recommended requirement for calcium is 1.2 grams daily. Eating this amount does not necessitate keeping a cow or goat in the backyard. To be sure, milk and milk products are the best sources of calcium. One glass (8 ounces) of milk contains about 0.3 grams of calcium, and so drinking four glasses a day will satisfy the calcium requirements of pregnancy. The nonmilk-drinking woman need not resort to bone meal as a source of calcium, however. Many people never drink milk as adults—some because of lactose intolerance[8] and others because of taste or tradition. Table 3 lists calcium-rich foods, most of which are suitable for those with lactose intolerance and which are likely to be

---

[8]Lactose intolerance refers to the inability to digest lactose, a sugar found in milk. This condition, which occurs in 80 to 90% of the world population, usually appears after early childhood and results in gastric distress after drinking milk. Dairy products made from the nonwatery part of milk, the curd (i.e., cheeses), can be eaten by lactose-intolerant people because most of the sugar is eliminated when these foods are made. Some parts of the country sell milk containing predigested lactose, called "acidopholus" milk, which can be drunk by those with lactose intolerance.

included at least occasionally in most people's diets (with one exception). The calcium content of foods not on the list can be determined by checking the food composition tables listed in Chapter 2. Other foods high in calcium include dandelion greens, kale, mustard greens, and beet greens. Because these vegetables are not consistently available in supermarkets or among the menu items in fast-food chains or vending machines, their utility as a source of calcium may be limited. Certain ethnic and regional groups in the United States do eat these foods regularly, a tradition that is to their nutritional advantage since these vegetables are also high in other nutrients, e.g., vitamin A and folic acid.

Many prepared foods contain calcium, especially those that include milk or milk products as an ingredient. If the pregnant woman consciously avoids all milk and dairy products, however, she may find it difficult to meet the calcium requirement of pregnancy unless she learns to include in her diet the nondairy sources of this mineral.

Folic Acid

A woman's need for folic acid *doubles* during pregnancy. This water-soluble vitamin and another (B_{12}) are used by multiplying cells to synthesize DNA (the repository of the cells' genetic information[9]). Since growth occurs only when new cells can be formed from older ones, these two vitamins, enabling this process to continue, are extremely important nutrients in fetal development. Vitamin B_{12} is found in numerous foods (meat, meat products, shellfish, fish, poultry, and dairy products) and resists destruction when food is cooked or processed; hence a deficiency of this nutrient is highly improbable with a normal diet. Even strict vegetarians may take years to develop a deficiency because the body is so careful about not wasting the vitamin B_{12} it has stored.

Folic acid occurs in almost all natural foods, so, theoretically, eating the recommended amount should be almost unavoidable. Unfortunately, though, this vitamin is very fragile; it can be destroyed easily by long cooking or by the temperatures used to can foods, and so its actual content in cooked or canned foods may be considerably less than when the food was in its original state. A pregnant woman has a crucial need for this vitamin since folic acid deficiency has been associated with serious complications of pregnancy, e.g., fetal damage and premature separation of the placenta at delivery.

Table 4 lists some folic acid-containing foods that are eaten occasionally in the American diet, as well as foods that are excellent sources of folic acid but are rarely eaten. Many other foods also contain this vitamin, but these are not listed because a person would have to consume huge quantities in order to obtain an appreciable amount of folic acid, thus rendering them impractical as sources of this nutrient.

---

[9]DNA contains the information that programs the producing of cellular protein through the use of an intermediary chemical, messenger RNA.

TABLE 4. *Folic acid content of some foods*

Food	Folic aicd (μg)
Common foods	
Cooked asparagus (4 spears)	436
Peanuts (4/5 cup)	257
Iceberg lettuce (¼ head)	25
Broccoli (2 spears)	154
Oatmeal (1 cup)	80
Cottage cheese (½ cup)	31
Spinach (½ cup)	67
Uncommon foods	
Lima beans (⅔ cup)	128
Mung bean sprouts (¾ cup)	145
Cowpeas (blackeye peas) (½ cup)	439
Raw beef liver[a] (3 oz)	294
Brewer's yeast (1 tbs)	162

[a]Unfortunately, only the folic acid content of raw liver is provided, probably because a variable amount is destroyed upon cooking; however, it is expected that the liver will be eaten cooked.

A quick calculation of the folic acid content of the "common foods" listed in Table 4 demonstrates the difficulty of eating the proper amount during pregnancy (unless you regularly eat asparagus or the "uncommon foods"). For this reason, physicians routinely advise their pregnant patients to take supplements containing folic acid.

Iron

Iron is another nutrient that must be obtained in significantly greater amounts during pregnancy. Iron forms part of the hemoglobin molecule (contained in red blood cells), which transports oxygen to the cells. As the circulatory system of the fetus develops, its quantity of blood and number of red blood cells increase. These processes require the formation of new hemoglobin and hence a continuous supply of additional iron. The fetus also stores iron during the gestational period to supply himself with enough iron to last 3 to 6 months after birth.

A pregnant woman's need for iron also increases because of demands made by her own body. The volume of her blood enlarges, in part because blood must be supplied to the placenta. In addition, some blood loss occurs during delivery. Although loss of iron from menstrual blood stops during pregnancy, the amount of iron saved does not compensate for the increased need, which can be more than double the amount required before pregnancy.

Female liver lovers probably enter pregnancy with adequate stores of iron and are relatively untouched by the iron demands of gestation. In contrast, women who eat a more typical American diet may be deficient in iron even before they become pregnant because of their monthly losses in menstrual blood. As much as

16 to 32 milligrams of iron can be lost each month; if this loss continues for several years without any compensation from the diet, a woman's stored iron will eventually be seriously depleted and severe anemia may result.

So many foods contain iron that a casual look at a food composition table seems to contradict the assertion that the average American diet is low in iron. However, this seems to be the case. To begin with, some of the iron-rich foods are rarely seen on the American dinner table, on restaurant menus, in airplanes, or in sandwich machines. Lima beans and liver, for example, are not ranked among the most frequently served foods in this country, and raw oysters are not within the price or taste range of many people. Although many other foods (e.g., vegetables, fruits, meats, and eggs) contain iron, two factors prevent the nutrient from being available to the body when these foods are eaten. First, the body normally absorbs only 2 to 10% of the iron in food (although absorption can increase when iron deficiency exists). Second, other compounds present in food may prevent iron from being transported across the intestinal wall into the circulation. For example, oatmeal contains a chemical that combines with the iron in the cereal to form a compound which cannot be absorbed by the body. Spinach, the Popeye superfood, contains substantial amounts of iron; but the iron in spinach and other green leafy vegetables is not absorbed well by the body, probably because of compounds (phytates) in these vegetables that attach to iron and prevent it from being transported into the circulation. The iron in eggs, another widely regarded source of this nutrient, is also absorbed poorly; only about 4% actually passes into the circulation.

The recommended daily iron intake is based on the assumption that about 10% of the ingested iron is actually absorbed, and consequently the number listed in the nutrition charts is 10 times higher than the amount the body needs. For a nonpregnant woman, the recommended daily allowance is 18 milligrams (mg); for the pregnant woman, it is 30 to 60 milligrams during the second and third trimesters.

The foods listed in Table 5 contain relatively high quantities of iron and, if eaten in sufficient amounts, can satisfy the daily iron requirement. The variety of such foods is limited, however, and many do not meet the average person's food preferences. For these reasons, physicians usually recommend iron supplements

TABLE 5. *Iron content of some foods*

Food	Iron (mg)
Beef liver (2 oz)	5.0
Lima beans (1 cup)	5.3
Tomato juice (1 cup)	2.2
Prune juice (1 cup)	10.5
Raisins (1 cup)	5.8
Bran flakes (40% bran) with added iron (1 cup)	12.3
Oysters (13–19 medium) (1 cup)	13.2
Hamburger (3 oz)	3.0

during pregnancy to ensure that their patients receive adequate amounts of this valuable nutrient.

EATING NUTRITIONALLY FOR TWO

Success in managing the nutritional aspect of prenatal care depends on the woman's eating habits before pregnancy. Some women have no difficulty adhering to the new nutritional dictates because the recommendations coincide with their current eating style. These are likely to be women who have been monitoring their food intake since they were 14, when, noticing a pimple or an extra pound, they decided to eliminate potato chips permanently from their diet. They can be recognized by their almost automatic inclusion of vegetables with any meal (except breakfast), their substitution of fruit for cake or pie at dessert time, and their vague uneasiness if a day goes by without citrus fruit or juice. Advising such a woman on the dietary modifications necessary for pregnancy is relatively simple. By analyzing her food intake over 4 or 5 days, she can detect any major deficiencies in her diet (it would be surprising to find any) and make minor substitutions in her normal food choices to meet the increased nutrient requirements of pregnancy. However, nutrients that she will need—particularly folic acid and iron—may require the use of supplements since these compounds are hard to obtain in sufficient amounts even from a "sensible" diet. This nutritionally knowledgeable woman will leave pregnancy behind with her nutrient stores relatively intact and will be prepared for the energy- and nutrient-consuming task of nursing her baby.

The nutritional care of the pregnant woman is not always so problem-free. There are several types of women for whom traditional dietary advice does not work. Since nutrient intake has such a major influence on the outcome of pregnancy, it is worth (a) examining the reasons why some types of nutritional management are not successful, and (b) exploring some alternate techniques.

The Pregnant Teenager

Of all pregnant women, the pregnant teenager (17 years old or younger) is the most vulnerable to the effects of an inadequate diet during pregnancy and the most difficult to convince of this fact. Her nutritional needs are greater than those of the adult because the nutritional cost of her own growth must be added to the requirements of the pregnancy itself. Unfortunately, of all women receiving prenatal care, she is probably the least receptive to nutritional advice. You cannot simply hand a pregnant teenager a list of foods and supplements and expect her to follow the recommendations. More intervention is needed because frequently the teenager, pregnant or not, has little interest in the nutritional aspects of food unless she can relate them to other elements of her life such as her appearance.

The pregnant teenager follows her peer group's eating style, which is, generally speaking, low in nutritional value. The diet of many teenage girls is deficient in calcium, vitamins A and C, iron, and thiamin (6). Should the pregnant teenager make no attempt to improve the quality of her diet, she may expose herself and her developing baby to serious nutritional deficiencies. Further complicating the nutritional quality of her diet is the rather common concern among this age group about weight gain and having a "nice" figure. As the pregnant teenager sees her shape changing with the advance of pregnancy, her response, quite frequently, is to reduce her food intake. Unfortunately, this decision to lose weight sometimes comes at the time of the most rapid fetal growth, and the young mother-to-be thus deprives herself and her baby of needed calories and nutrients. Other factors (e.g., problems at home, lack of money for supplements, or the need to live away from home) may also affect the pregnant teenager's diet, and traditional approaches to nutritional counseling do not have a high success rate among these girls. Convincing an adolescent that what she eats will influence the outcome of her pregnancy is difficult, especially if the suggested diet differs radically from the foods she likes and is accustomed to eating. (How many of us, knowing that a piece of pie or cake today will affect our weight tomorrow, can modify our immediate desire for that particular food? It is even harder if the result of our food choice will not be visible for 6 to 9 months and if our immediate concern is to maintain our figure at all costs.)

Therefore the mere teaching of nutritional theory will probably not affect the teenager's food choices. A nurse relates her experience in conducting nutrition classes for a group of pregnant girls:

> Each class, held at noon, was dutifully attended by all of the girls going to the obstetrical clinic. They listened attentively while eating lunch. These, unfortunately, were always the same—soft drinks and potato chips!

Perhaps advertising is the only method by which this age group (pregnant or not) can be convinced that eating has a direct affect on their health and that of their babies. If magazines for the female teenage population can display an assortment of cosmetics containing a refrigerator's worth of fruits and vegetables (apricot handcream, cucumber shampoo, avocado eye shadow), then advertising could also promote such food for use *inside* the body. Considering the high risk of pregnancy complications among this age group (6, 7), as well as the possible insult to the mother's growth and health, these young women should be educated on sound prenatal nutrition through the media that have been most successful in influencing other aspects of their lifestyle.

The Pregnant Poor

Economic factors can also affect the nutritional status of a woman and her baby. Pregnant women whose diets are nutritionally inferior because of lack of money are probably eating the same foods they ate before becoming pregnant. Their limited food choices frequently do not supply enough of the nutrients considered essential for maintenance of a healthy pregnancy. These women often enter pregnancy with marginal nutrient reserves (anemia from iron insufficiency is quite common); the added nutrient burden of pregnancy without an accompanying improvement in their diet can affect the pregnancy. In addition to insufficient intake of iron and occasionally animal protein, the pregnant poor do not obtain enough folic acid, vitamin A, and often calcium in their diets.

Sometimes good sources of these nutrients are neglected not because of price but because they are unacceptable to certain ethnic or regional groups: Many of the nutrients are unfamiliar to people who move from one geographic region to another and who can no longer find the same fruits, vegetables, and cereal grains they were used to eating; these foods may also be rejected for reasons of taste, religion, or health. (A pregnant woman with lactose intolerance is unlikely to drink four glasses of milk a day. Unless someone carefully indicates alternate sources of calcium to her, she may not obtain enough of this nutrient in her diet.)

In many cases, available cash, which could purchase vitamin and mineral supplements or certain foods recommended by a physician, is spent instead on food for the entire family or on items that have higher priority for the limited money on hand. The WIC program, discussed previously, seems to deal successfully with some of these problems because it makes money available for specific food items that will fill the nutritional gaps in the woman's regular diet. The use of this program, plus nutritional counseling to help the woman integrate valuable foods into her eating style, can have a positive effect on the nutritional success of her pregnancy.

Other Groups

A woman does not have to be poor to eat poorly. She may go through pregnancy with access to the "proper" diet and money for vitamin and mineral supplements and yet be inadequately nourished. The following sections describe briefly some other categories of pregnant women whose diets may be incompatible with good nutrition.

Nutritionally Negligent Individual

The nutritionally negligent woman pays little attention to the nutritional quality of her diet. Nutrition has a very low priority among the factors motivating her food choices, and she may be deficient in one or more nutrients primarily because she neglects to include the foods that supply these nutrients. Her food choices are likely to be influenced by whim or convenience, and she is probably unaware of her diet's nutritional content. If this woman works away from home and depends on restaurants, sandwich shops, and vending machines for one or two of her daily meals, she may be obtaining only marginal amounts of certain vitamins and minerals from the foods available to her (see Chapter 1). If she continues to work during her pregnancy, she may have to adjust her eating habits rather strenuously in order to meet the increased nutritional demands of her body.

Handing the negligent eater a diet plan that lists servings of green, red, and yellow vegetables along with required amounts of milk and meat is unlikely to effect any permanent change in her eating habits. She may be willing to follow the plan for a few weeks, but only a strongly motivated person will continue to modify her eating for as long as 8 or 9 months. (Consider how difficult it is to follow any kind of diet for longer than 2 weeks, especially if it entails a major alteration in eating habits.) This type of eater needs help in (a) acquiring insight into her regular eating habits, and (b) changing her food choices so her nutritional needs are met without conflicting with her accustomed lifestyle.

Frequently Pregnant Woman

A woman who goes through several closely spaced pregnancies may risk the development of greater nutritional deficiencies with each succeeding pregnancy. If she followed an inadequate diet during one pregnancy and did not improve her food choices afterward, she will enter her subsequent pregnancies with marginal stores of various nutrients. If this cycle of poor food choices during and between pregnancies continues, the woman risks severe deficiencies for herself and her baby.

This situation can occur even when a woman's diet is not obviously inadequate. Often such a woman eats poorly simply because she does not spend time thinking about what she should be eating. She attends to the dietary needs of her children, worries about whether they are getting enough vitamins and minerals, and even buys vitamin pills for the family because "no one eats any vegetables." However, while urging her children to drink their milk, eat their liver, and chew their carrots, the same woman breakfasts on leftover toast, eats leftover baby food or peanut butter and jelly sandwiches for lunch, and prepares supper with foods the family likes without regard for her own nutritional needs. After her third, fourth, or fifth pregnancy, a woman has often grown indifferent to her own requirements and believes that she need not worry about taking care of herself during *this* pregnancy since all the others went so well.

One cannot assume, therefore, that a woman who has gone through many pregnancies is knowledgeable about the diet she should follow and will make wise food choices, or that she will conscientiously take the recommended vitamin and mineral supplements. These women should be advised of their nutritional needs regardless of the number of previous pregnancies, and they should be offered the additional admonition that a good diet need not stop after the baby is born!

Ideological Eater

Women who follow ideologically prescribed eating patterns may be unable or unwilling to alter their food choices in order to obtain the nutrients recommended for pregnancy. Vegetarians, who may eliminate eggs and dairy products as well as meat and fish from their diets, or members of the macrobiotic community, whose diet consists primarily of grains and vegetables, may not be able to obtain the required amounts of protein, iron, or calcium from the limited variety of foods they eat. If a woman following an ideological diet also does not believe in taking vitamin and mineral supplements, her diet may be inadequate to support a healthy pregnancy. Often, however, only slight modifications are necessary to provide the diet with missing nutrients (choosing the proper combinations of vegetable protein, for example, or eating more calcium-rich vegetables such as kale or mustard greens).

Some ideological diets promote the ingestion of large quantities of certain vitamins, e.g., vitamins C or A. Pregnant women who take excessive doses of vitamin supplements (perhaps a thousand times the recommended amount) may be exposing their developing fetuses to potential nutritional deficiencies after birth or congenital malformations. Some animal studies (8) provide evidence that excessive vitamin C intake by the pregnant animal may increase the vitamin C requirement of its offspring and thereby render the young animal more susceptible to vitamin C deficiency (during the first month of its life) than an animal whose mother received normal amounts of vitamin C during pregnancy. Excessive ingestion of vitamin A by a pregnant rabbit can produce developmental malformations in its offspring, and current studies indicate that other animal species, perhaps including humans, may respond in a similar fashion (8–10). Therefore a diet that includes excessive amounts of various nutrients can be potentially harmful to the fetus and should be avoided by the pregnant woman.

COMMENT

Babies are not made from coal, water, and air, but rather from the organic and inorganic materials we call nutrients. The mother is the ultimate source of these substances. Her own reserves and her diet continuously supply nutrients to the developing fetus. Although sporadic dietary indulgences (an occasional hot fudge sundae) have little effect on the outcome of the pregnancy (although some impact on the woman's fat stores), a consistent intake of nutrients in the recommended quantities is essential to ensure a healthy baby and mother.

REFERENCES

1. Seifrit, E. (1968): Changes in beliefs and food practices in pregnancy. In: *Lydia J. Roberts Award Essays,* pp. 79–90. American Dietetic Association, Chicago.
2. Committee on Maternal Nutrition (1970): *Maternal Nutrition and the Course of Pregnancy: Summary Report.* National Academy of Sciences, Washington, D.C.
3. Baker, H., Frank, O., Thomson, A., Langer, A., Munves, E., de Angelis, B., and Kaminetisky, H. (1975): Vitamin profile of 174 mothers and newborns at parturition. *Am. J. Clin. Nutr.,* 28:56–65.
4. National Academy of Sciences (1979): *Recommended Dietary Allowances,* 9th ed. National Academy of Sciences, Washington, D.C. *(in press).*
5. Lechtig, A., Yarbrough, C., Delgados, H., Habicht, J-P., Matorell, R., and Klein, R. (1975): Influence of maternal nutrition on birth weight. *Am. J. Clin. Nutr.,* 28:1225–1233.

6. Shank, R. (1970): Maternal nutrition. *Nutr. Today,* 5:1–13.
7. Department of Health, Education, and Welfare (1970): *Ten-State Nutrition Survey.* DHEW Publication No. 72-8134. Government Printing Office, Washington, D.C.
8. Norkis, E., and Rosso, P. (1975): Changes in ascorbic acid metabolism of the offspring following high maternal intake of this vitamin in the pregnant guinea pig. *Ann. N.Y. Acad. Sci.* 258:401–409.
9. Kochar, D.M., and Johnson, E.M. (1965): Morphological and autoradiographic studies of cleft palate induced in rat embryos by maternal hypervitaminosis A. *J. Embryol. Exp. Morphol.,* 223:238.
10. Gal, I., Sharman, I., Pryse, J., and Davies, J. (1972): Vitamin A in relation to human congenital malformations. *Adv. Teratol.,* 5:143–159.

6 THE NEW EATER: Nutrition During Infancy

Feeding the infant has two effects: It provides the nutrients necessary for rapid growth and development, and it gives the infant the associations, memories, and emotions that later become part of his[1] own style of eating. Supplying the nutrients is the simple part of feeding the infant. Structuring an "eating environment" that will develop rational and nutritionally sound eating behavior is, at best, only partially successful, as illustrated by the almost universal preference of young children for a cookie over a carrot. Both aspects of infant feeding are discussed in this chapter, along with previous theories of infant feeding, current infant feeding fashions, and an evaluation of the breast-feeding/bottle-feeding controversy. In addition, the chapter includes nutritional information for the mother who chooses to breast-feed her baby.

PAST METHODS OF CHILD FEEDING

The infant and child feeding practices of the past reflected an almost total ignorance of the effect of nutrition on growth and development. For example, a baby today is fed supplemental food by 6 months of age or earlier since it is now recognized that milk alone cannot provide enough calories or nutrients for the infant's growth beyond 6 months. Babies fed only milk after this age grow more slowly and are usually smaller than babies whose diets are supplemented with baby food. Yet even at the beginning of this century, physicians recommended that weaning (feeding baby food in addition to milk) be delayed until at least four teeth could be seen in the baby's mouth (usually around 8 to 12 months of age) (1).

The foods selected for weaning made as little nutritional sense as the delay. The most common weaning foods were pap, a concoction of flour or bread cooked in water, and panada, a flour, cereal, or bread-crumb mixture cooked in broth or milk. These thick, gelatinous, porridge-type foods supplied calories to the baby's diet but little else. Fruits and vegetables were not given to the child until the second or third year because they were thought to cause infantile diarrhea, which was common and often fatal. Since the value of these foods in providing vitamins and minerals was not recognized until this century, eliminating them from the diet was not considered nutritionally harmful. Beef tea or beef gruel were often fed to young children, but meat itself was offered only sparingly. Until this century, meat was generally withheld from children's diets until age 3 because it was thought to

---

[1]The pronoun "he" is used to represent babies of both sexes simply because it is easier to use one term—and "he" is easier to spell than "she"!

be indigestible. On the other hand, milk was not fed to the child after weaning because it was not considered appropriate for anyone but a nursing baby. Eggs, however,were allowed and, along with cereals, puddings, and broths, comprised most of the child's foods until 2 to 3 years of age.

Although it is obvious to us that such a limited diet must have deprived the child of nutrients needed for growth, the idea that food contains nutrients that support growth and maintain health has developed only during the last 100 years. This concept had to precede the selection of a diet that contained nutrients to meet the infant's specific needs. Moreover, the child's need for sufficient energy (calories) was not well understood until this century, and children were often given too little food. (Children in English boarding schools were deliberately fed too little because it kept them quiet.)

One often hears the statement that children grow bigger today than in the past because they are better nourished. Although this statement is true, we are rarely told that children could have been better nourished in the past had the feeding practices of the time allowed them to eat the foods available.

Infants were even more vulnerable to seemingly arbitrary modes of feeding than older children. A common belief for many centuries was that colostrum (the milk-like substance produced by the mother before true milk secretion) was bad for a newborn (2). The mother was not allowed to nurse until her "milk came in"; instead, newborns were sometimes hand-fed a mixture of butter and sugar or oil, panada, or crackers ground up in gruel (1).

If the mother was unable to nurse at all, the infant was either given to a wet nurse, fed cow's milk, or given a mixture of bread and milk. Wet nurses often took care of many babies at the same time; unsupervised and often negligent, they caused many infants to die from disease or starvation. Artificially fed babies were no better off than those entrusted to a wet nurse. Cow's milk was fed undiluted to young infants, even though its protein and mineral composition is much greater than that of human milk. (By the end of the nineteenth century, the difference in composition was recognized, and the milk was diluted with water for infant feeding.) Undiluted cow's milk was hard for babies to digest, and its high mineral and protein content often caused problems. In addition, milk was frequently contaminated because dairies were filthy, and no control was maintained over the condition of the cows or the handling of the milk. Bottles with nipples are a recent innovation; earlier devices, usually consisting of a soft rag tied to the end of a nozzle or spout of a can, did not work very well. Both the container and rag were sources of contamination—if the baby did not become sick from the contaminated milk, he risked infection from the contaminated feeding device. The mortality rate for artificially fed infants was even higher than for those fed by a wet nurse. Some babies were fed only pap or gruel, and these children never survived.

Once nutrition became a science and the role of specific nutrients in the growth and maintenance of the baby was understood, infant feeding practices left the Dark Ages and began to promote, rather than impair, the health of the child.

The baby has "come a long way," thanks to improvements in infant feeding practices. The change in the quality of nutritional care was due, in part, to simultaneous advances in the science of nutrition and the new technology of food processing. Baby foods and milk formulas were produced free from contamination relatively inexpensively and with nutrients appropriate for the baby and young child. These developments made possible children's survival through infancy and their optimal growth and development.

NUTRIENT NEEDS OF THE INFANT

Nutrient needs of the infant are based on their requirements for growth, a phenomenon that occurs continuously throughout childhood. This process evokes great wonder in grandparents, who inevitably exclaim, "My how he/she has grown!" when viewing the grandchild after an interval of some weeks or months. Growing, however, is common and normal for a child. When growth does not occur at a normal rate, the child is described as "failing to thrive," and the reasons must be investigated.

The infant needs nutrients for two purposes: to fulfill the daily maintenance requirements of his body and to promote the growth and development of new tissue. (Adults need nutrients only for maintenance, unless they are rapidly developing new muscle or replacing injured tissue.)

Protein

During the first 4 months of a baby's life, more than half of the protein consumed is used to form new tissue. Scientific estimates of the protein requirements of infants are remarkably close to the actual protein content of human milk.[2] Commercial infant formula contains about 20% more protein than human milk to ensure that infants who are unable to utilize the protein in cow's milk as efficiently as that in human milk will obtain sufficient protein. (Some of the protein in a formula may not be absorbed into the blood during digestion and instead passes out of the body in the feces.)

Like adults, infants depend on dietary protein for essential amino acids (amino acids are the basic components of protein), since they cannot be made by the body.[3] Not surprisingly, the pattern of essential amino acids in human milk comes close to meeting the infant's amino acid requirements.

To the amazement of many mothers and grandmothers, many pediatricians believe that an infant's requirement for protein and other nutrients can be supplied totally by human milk, formula, or cow's milk until the infant is about 6 months old. (However, pediatricians usually recommend feeding vitamin and iron supplements along with the milk.) Bowing to park bench pressure, doctors permit

---

[2]Human milk contains 1.1 grams of protein in every 100 milliliters, and 1.5 grams of protein for every 100 calories.

[3]The essential amino acids are: valine, isoleucine, leucine, lysine, threonine, tryptophan, phenylalanine, methionine, and histidine.

or recommend that babies be started on some baby food considerably before that age (more on this later in the chapter). Strained cereals and fruit are usually the baby's first "real" foods, although they are largely carbohydrate and contain considerably less protein than milk. Moreover, the essential amino acid composition of the protein in these foods is not matched to the baby's requirements; for example, some essential amino acids (e.g., tryptophan) are not contained in sufficient amounts for the baby's needs. If the young infant is fed so much low-protein baby food that his milk consumption drops significantly, he may not be obtaining sufficient amounts of high-quality protein.[4] Adding cereal or strained fruit to the milk bottle can cause the same problem. (This trick is used to avoid sticky "banana buildup" on mother after each feeding.) The bulk of the milk plus cereal in the bottle may fill the baby before he has drunk enough milk to satisfy his protein needs. For a young baby, therefore, a little baby food is better than a lot.

Calories

A baby's body uses about 7.5 calories to make 1 gram of protein and about 11.5 calories for 1 gram of fat (4). During the first 4 months of life, approximately one-third of the infant's caloric intake goes toward the formation of new tissue. After 4 months he begins to grow less rapidly, and the percentage of calories needed for growth also decreases. Between the fourth and twelfth months, 7.4% of the calories in his diet are used for growth; this percentage decreases to 1.6% between the first and second years of life, and to 1% between the second and third years.

The baby's activity level also affects his energy needs. A baby who constantly rolls around the changing table or squirms all over his grandmother's lap probably uses more calories than the placid, Buddha-like infant who stares disinterestedly at the passing scene when not taking long naps. Crying contributes to caloric need; a baby uses 100% more calories when crying than when content.

Accurately translating a particular baby's activity level into specific caloric needs is difficult. The mother is generally the best qualified to define and describe her baby's activity, and her information will enable the baby's doctor to determine how much food he should be eating.

Milk is the primary source of energy for the baby. Human milk contains 65 to 75 calories in 100 milliliters (3.5 ounces); commercial milk-based formulas are similar. As infants grow, the amount of milk they drink increases. If we divide the number of calories an infant eats each day by his weight, then for a given weight the infant consumes the most calories between the second and fourth weeks of life (4). A bottle-fed baby's weight and, to some extent, activity determine the amount of milk he should be given; a breast-fed baby will consume what he needs by the duration and frequency of nursing. Although bottle-fed babies drink greater total

---

[4]The difference between the protein content of baby cereal and milk is considerable (3). A jar of strained rice cereal with apples and bananas contains about 93 calories and 0.5 grams of protein, whereas a volume of human milk containing 100 calories has about 1.5 to 1.7 grams of protein, and commercial formula (same calories) about 2.2 to 2.7 grams of protein.

quantities of milk as they grow, their requirements in terms of body weight decrease: for the first month, they usually drink about 3 ounces of formula for each pound; after that, they need only about 1.5 ounces per pound.

Parents and grandparents sometimes decide they know better than the baby how much milk he should be drinking and so coax him to "finish the bottle." Several studies indicate that babies are capable of adjusting the amount of milk they drink to meet their own caloric needs by the time they are 40 days old (4). In one study, babies were fed milk with the appropriate number of calories for their age, and the amount they drank was compared with the amount consumed by babies fed milk containing twice as many calories in the same volume. After a few weeks, all the babies, who were now about 40 days old, were consuming the same number of calories—the babies fed the high-calorie milk simply drank less.

Fat

Fat provides the infant with energy and two essential fatty acids (arachidonic and linoleic acids). The fat in human milk and commercial infant formula can be digested easily; butterfat, the fat in cow's milk, is not so readily absorbed by the young baby, and the unabsorbed portion is eliminated in the feces. When fat is lost through elimination, the baby must increase his food consumption to compensate. According to some pediatricians, switching the baby from human milk or formula to cow's milk before a large portion of his calories come from baby food may be risky since a baby cannot absorb enough butterfat to meet his caloric needs. Waiting until the baby consumes about two jars of strained baby food daily, or the equivalent in home-prepared food (about 1 cup or 8 ounces), ensures that another source of calories is available to him should butterfat absorption from milk be inefficient.

Skim milk is not an acceptable substitute for whole milk for the young infant, although it is recommended for children over 2 years of age (4). Skim milk provides the infant with four times more protein than he needs but insufficient amounts of fat (calories) and essential fatty acids.[5]

The practice of substituting skim milk for formula or whole milk (when the child is old enough to drink it) is popular among mothers and some pediatricians who wish to prevent babies from becoming fat! Babies as young as 4 to 6 months are being fed skim milk, even though it is almost impossible for a baby of this age to drink a large enough quantity of skim milk to obtain the number of calories needed for growth (4). A leading pediatrician and nutritionist, Dr. Samuel Fomon, warns that feeding skim milk to a young baby may cause him to used stored fat for some of his energy requirements (4). Should the baby then become sick and stop eating

---

[5]Some types of skim milk, however, contain 2% butterfat (about half as much as whole milk) and provide only slightly more protein and less fat than human milk, formula, or cow's milk. Although no undesirable consequences have yet been detected with this type of milk, no desirable ones have been found either.

for some time, he might not have sufficient stored fat for his energy needs during this period.

The current trend of feeding skim milk to babies is motivated by the belief that "lean" children will be less vulnerable to heart disease in later life.[6]

Are the proponents of low-fat diets for infants correct? Since we cannot wait 25 or 30 years to find out if infants fed skim milk grow up to be skinny adults with fat-free arteries, a look at infant feeding practices of the past may give us some insight into the question.

Until this century, breast-fed infants were not weaned until 18 to 24 months of age, a practice still followed in many developing countries. Although some soft, cereal-like food may have been offered to these infants, milk was the major source of calories and nutrients.

The fat content of milk increases with the length of the lactation period (5, 6). After 2 years of nursing, a mother's milk contains twice as much fat as it contained after 1 month of nursing (5, 6). An anthropologist who analyzed the milk of nursing mothers from a Bushmen tribe in Africa noted that the milk from a woman who had nursed for over 3 years resembled whipping cream, and indeed her milk contained five times as much fat as milk from other women in the same village who had nursed for 18 months or less.

When milk is the primary food of a 2- or 3-year-old child, the high fat (and thus caloric) content becomes critically important in fulfilling the child's caloric needs. Compare this natural phenomenon—the older the nursing baby, the more fat he receives in the milk—with the contemporary recommendation: the older the baby, the less fat he receives from milk. Of course, almost all babies in our society are eating foods other than milk by 2 to 3 years of age (usually by 2 to 3 months), so the caloric content of milk is not critical for their health and growth. No one would suggest to a nursing mother in our society that she stop nursing after a year or so because the fat content of her milk might be unacceptably high; she might be told, however, to feed her child skim milk once breast feeding is discontinued because its low fat content is better for the baby. The composition of breast milk has had one major effect; it has ensured the survival of the human race. We do not know what the effect of altering the composition of milk will be, and we cannot wait several thousand years to find out. Perhaps human milk should remain the standard.

Carbohydrate

About 30% to 40% of the calories in milk come from carbohydrate, which is present in milk as the sugar lactose.[7] In the intestine, lactose is split into its two

---

[6]It has been suggested that decreasing an infant's consumption of fat lowers his cholesterol intake, and this in turn decreases the accumulation of fat along the walls of his arteries. However, no conclusive evidence is available to support this theory.

[7]Lactose is a type of sugar called a disaccharide because it is composed of two sugar units, glucose and galactose. It tastes less sweet than sucrose (table sugar), which is why we do not think of milk as a sweet food.

sugar components (glucose and galactose) by an enzyme[8] (lactase), and each sugar unit is absorbed into the bloodstream. The amount of lactase diminishes with age, however, and many older children and adults are unable to digest lactose completely. This is an extremely common condition known as lactose intolerance.[9] People who are lactose-intolerant simply do not have much of the enzyme when they reach school age or older and usually, almost unconsciously, decrease their milk consumption at that time. Infants, however, rarely suffer from lactose intolerance.

The lactose in milk is an indirect cause of dental caries (cavities) because it promotes the growth of bacteria. Babies who suck at a bottle of formula or milk while falling asleep may develop "nursing bottle syndrome." This condition is characterized by badly decayed primary teeth, especially in the upper front of the mouth, where the teeth are bathed in milk almost continuously. Tooth decay of this type is produced to an even greater extent when the baby is allowed to fall asleep while sucking a bottle filled with fruit juice, a sweetened artificial fruit drink, or soft drink. The sugar content of these drinks promotes rapid growth of bacteria in the mouth.[10]

Most baby foods contain a great deal of carbohydrates: starch, sugar, or both. Egg yolks, strained meats, and dinners rich in meat are exceptions. Sucrose or dextrose are often added to puddings, creamed vegetables, fruits, fruit juices, and deserts because babies like the taste of sweet foods. (Putting a dollop of applesauce or banana on a teaspoon of spinach or liver is a traditional way of getting baby to try the food, but some babies are clever enough to lick off the applesauce and spit out the spinach.)

The addition of sugar to baby foods has been criticized by many parents who feel that exposing the baby to sweet foods will cause him to develop a "sweet tooth." Although it would be comforting to blame an adult addiction for chocolate chips on an excess of strained applesauce during babyhood, scientific evidence simply does not support this relationship. Many research studies have demonstrated an almost universal preference for a sweet-tasting drink over a bland solution (e.g., water) among very young animals and babies. One scientist tested his own newborn daughter for taste preference and found that she preferred a sweet solution when she was only a few hours old (7).

Recently our laboratory conducted an experiment in which we fed three groups of suckling rats either (a) a small amount of a sweet-tasting strained baby cereal containing fruit; (b) milk; or (c) water. After the rats were weaned, all three groups were given a choice between a sweet- or a bland-tasting food. If exposing one group to the sweet-tasting baby cereal while they were still nursing would develop

---

[8]Enzymes are proteins that speed up chemical reactions.

[9]About 80% of the world's population is lactose-intolerant; European Caucasians are among the few groups able to tolerate milk in large quantities as adults.

[10]Sucrose (table sugar) is made up to two simple sugars, glucose and fructose, and is probably the most efficient sugar for promoting tooth decay.

a sweet tooth in them but not in the others, we would expect to find a decided preference for the sweet weaning food among that group. We found, however, that all the baby rats, regardless of what they had been fed previously, preferred the sweet food to the bland, and that this preference persisted until they were almost mature animals.

Although the baby does not need the extra calories contributed by the added sucrose, it seems unlikely that feeding a sweet-tasting preparation to a baby causes him to develop a preference for sweets. If the mother always smiles as she feeds the baby the sweet-tasting bananas and unconsciously makes a face as she spoons out the spinach or strained liver, the baby might learn to associate sweets with a maternal smile and nonsweet food with a facial grimace. Hence these early experiences may contribute to an adult's preference for chocolate chips over liver.

Starch is added to many baby foods to prevent the watery portion of the food from separating out and forming a puddle on top. Starch contributes no nutritional value to the food except calories, and pediatricians have questioned whether some of the starch added to strained baby food can be properly digested by infants. The reason for adding starch is aesthetic; the food looks better and may even feel better in the mouth. A similar effect could probably be achieved by vigorous stirring with a spoon. Thickening baby food with additional amounts of the major ingredients (noodles and chicken, apples, bananas), instead of starch, would give the food greater nutritional value.

Vitamins and Minerals

Human milk or commercial formula supplies most of the infant's vitamin and mineral needs. As the baby grows, his increasing needs can be met by baby foods—especially cereals, vegetables, fruits, and meat preparations—and cow's milk. Table 1 lists the vitamin and mineral requirements of the infant at various ages up to 36 months.

Vitamin A is abundant in the average American child's diet. Milk and infant formula contain sufficient amounts of this vitamin to meet the nursing baby's needs; eggs, meat, dairy products, and yellow and green vegetables (winter squash, carrots, spinach, broccoli) constitute an additional source once the child can eat a variety of solid foods. Because this vitamin is so plentiful in the infant's diet, physicians tend to worry more about the danger of excess vitamin A (through the misuse of vitamin supplements) than the danger of vitamin A deficiency. As Table 1 shows, the daily requirement for vitamin A is the same for a 12-month-old as for a 36-month-old child (2,000 IU). Cases have been reported of infants receiving 10 times that amount (20,000 IU) and developing symptoms of vitamin A toxicity: loss of skin cells, increased pressure on the brain, and loss of appetite. (Although many adults consume excessive amounts of the vitamin, their larger size may prevent toxic effects.) The mother who carefully follows her pediatrician's instructions, however, is not likely to give her child an overdose of vitamin A.

TABLE 1. *Recommended daily intakes of vitamins and minerals at age 0 to 36 months*

Nutrient	0–6 Months	6–12 Months	12–36 Months
Vitamins			
A (IU)	1,400	2,000	2,000
D (IU)	400	400	400
E (IU)	4	5	7
C (mg)	60	60	65
Folic acid (μg)	50	50	100
Niacin (mg)	5	8	9
Riboflavin (mg)	0.4	0.6	0.8
Thiamin (mg)	0.3	0.5	0.7
B_6 (mg)	0.3	0.4	0.6
B_{12} (mg)	0.3	0.3	1.0
Minerals			
Calcium (mg)	360	540	800
Phosphorus (mg)	240	400	800
Iodine (μg)	35	45	60
Iron (mg)	10	15	15
Magnesium (mg)	60	70	150
Zinc (mg)	3	5	10

From ref. 15.
IU = international units; mg = milligrams; μg = micrograms.

Vitamin D

Cod liver oil, an excellent source of vitamin D, was often fed to infants and older children, its taste barely masked by the orange juice in which it was usually dissolved. Until recently pediatricians' offices often smelled of cod liver oil because its odor permeated the cushions and curtains of waiting rooms. Cod liver oil is still given to the breast-fed infant, along with less smelly forms of vitamin D, because human milk does not contain sufficient amounts of this vitamin to meet the baby's needs (400 IU daily). Commercial infant formula and cow's milk are fortified with enough vitamin D to make supplementation unnecessary.

The human body can manufacture vitamin D. When the skin is exposed to sunlight or artificial ultraviolet light of a particular wavelength, a substance in the skin is changed to vitamin D. Theoretically, vitamin D supplements should be unnecessary since sunbathing ought to fulfill the baby's needs. However, cold winters, hot summers, and modesty tend to reduce the amount of time the skin is exposed to the sun, and dietary supplements must also be relied on.

Vitamin D is involved in the absorption of calcium from the small intestine into the circulatory system. The vitamin regulates the production of protein, which transports calcium from the intestine to the cells from which it enters the bloodstream. Since calcium is needed for the formation of bones and teeth, which develop rapidly in the young child, vitamin D has a crucial function during this period.

Vitamins E and K

Vitamins E and K are adequately supplied in breast milk and commercial formula. Since human milk contains less vitamin K than formula, pediatricians often give the newborn supplemental vitamin K if the mother plans to breast-feed. (Vitamin K is involved in the multistep process of blood clotting, and a deficiency of this vitamin can cause internal bleeding.) As the quantity of milk the infant drinks increases, the intake of this vitamin will also increase, making additional supplementation unnecessary.

Vitamin C

Human milk contains enough vitamin C for the infant, but cow's milk does not; commercial formulas made from cow's milk are therefore fortified with this vitamin. Fresh cow's milk contains considerable vitamin C, but processing procedures such as pasteurization destroy most of the vitamin. About 100 years ago physicians recommended that mothers boil cow's milk before feeding it to their babies because this procedure seemed to decrease the incidence of bacterial diseases among young children. After boiling milk became common, physicians noted that the babies were no longer dying of infantile diarrhea; instead, they died of scurvy. Eventually, physicians realized that vitamin C is destroyed after prolonged boiling, and its absence in the diet causes scurvy.

Until fairly recently, milk was the only reliable source of vitamin C for infants and young children living in northern climates, since fruits and vegetables were available only during certain seasons and even then were rarely fed to young children. Since boiling milk destroyed organisms that made children sick, a dilemma arose that was not solved until synthetic vitamin C became available.

Most children today are accustomed to eating a variety of foods rich in vitamin C by the time cow's milk is substituted for formula. As the child grows and develops a more selective palate, however, he may avoid foods containing vitamin C. The child who associates orange only with crayons, who may not tolerate citrus juices very well, and who carefully throws all vegetables on the floor can successfully avoid all contact with this vitamin. Vitamin C is plentiful when the correct foods are eaten (citrus fruits and their juices, baked potato, cabbage, tomato, dark green leafy vegetables, green pepper) but is easy to overlook on a limited diet.

B Vitamins

Thiamin, riboflavin, niacin, pyridoxine, and folic acid are supplied in amounts adequate for the infant's needs in human and cow's milk as well as in commercial formulas. Niacin is also made by the body from tryptophan, an essential amino acid that must be obtained in the diet.

Milk or formula also fulfills an infant's requirement for vitamin B_{12}. This vitamin is found only in foods of animal origin. A strictly vegetarian diet (no eggs, milk, dairy products, meat, or fish) will fail to provide a young child with the amount he requires after weaning and a B_{12} supplement should be given.[11]

Minerals

The body uses a variety of minerals, which must be supplied in the diet. Some of the major minerals are sodium, potassium, chloride, phosphorus, magnesium, sulfur, and iron. Others, called trace minerals, sound more like a list of ingredients for a bag of fertilizer: copper, zinc, chromium, nickel, manganese, molybdenum, cadmium, cobalt, and selenium. Although specific requirements for some of these trace minerals have not yet been established, all are needed by the body. They participate in various chemical activities in the cells and are integrated into the structural components of the body as well, e.g., the skeletal system. For example, magnesium participates in the chemical reactions that produce adenosine triphosphate (ATP), a substance in body cells that stores energy within its chemical structure. Magnesium is also involved in the transfer of energy from ATP to the chemical substances involved in synthetic activities in the cells, e.g., protein formation. (Magnesium binds messenger RNA to ribosomes, the cellular structures on which proteins are made.)

Most of the minerals eaten by the infant are used for the formation of new tissue. Small amounts go to replace the minerals excreted daily in the urine, feces, and sweat. Except for iron, minerals are supplied in sufficient quantity in human and cow's milk and infant formula.

One mineral, sodium, may be too well supplied in the diet. It is eaten in the form of salt; and although its content in milk is compatible with the baby's needs, individually salted or processed baby foods may contain more than is needed or desirable. Too much salt in the diet has been implicated in the development of hypertension, a disease characterized by high blood pressure. Physicians caution everyone to limit salt intake, especially those with a family history of this disease. Babies therefore should not be exposed to large quantities of salt, and baby food companies have recently reduced the salt content of prepared baby food. Mothers and other people feeding a bland-tasting strained preparation to an infant are tempted to add salt. Salting the food, however, may result in an unacceptably high sodium intake for the baby. Mothers who prepare homemade baby food by grinding up the family's food should be careful about this.

> An acquaintance preparing food for her 5-month-old son in my kitchen recently illustrated this point. She brought with her pots, carrots, potatoes, meat, broth, and a food grinder. As she boiled, mashed, ground, and stirred the food, she lectured me on the virtues of homemade, "additive-free" baby food. Her preparations over, she dumped the mush into a feeding dish, tasted a small amount, muttered, "it needs salt," and shook a copious amount into the food. Clearly, she did not regard adding salt to her own taste as potentially harmful for her baby.

Calcium and phosphorus are minerals of critical and continuous importance to

---

[11]A strictly vegetarian nursing mother may produce milk with insufficient B_{12} content. She should ask her pediatrician about a B_{12} supplement for herself or her infant.

the growing baby because of their major roles in the formation of the skeleton. Throughout childhood these and most of the other minerals are amply supplied by milk and other dairy products unless the child is not allowed to eat these foods for ideological or medical reasons. Eliminating dairy products from the diet, as in vegetarian or macrobiotic diets (see Chapter 2), may severely reduce the amount of calcium the child receives. Calcium deficiency and growth retardation may result unless the child is provided with adequate substitutes, e.g., dark green leafy vegetables (kale, mustard greens, beet greens).

Iron is an essential component of hemoglobin, the substance in red blood cells that binds oxygen. It also forms part of a muscle protein (myoglobulin) and attaches to specific enzymes in the cells. Red blood cells live about 120 days and are replaced continually by new ones synthesized in the bone marrow. Most of the iron in an adult's diet is used to make hemoglobin for new red blood cells; iron recycled from the "dead" cells is also used for this purpose. Infants and young children require iron not only to replace existing red blood cells but also for the formation of new red blood cells, cellular enzymes, and muscle protein during growth.

Babies are born with a supply of iron that theoretically should meet their needs for 2 to 3 months. However, since even well-nourished mothers can give birth to babies with inadequate iron stores, many pediatricians feel that a baby should start getting iron either in the diet or in a vitamin-mineral supplement by 1 month of age. Many formulas are fortified with iron, and so long as the baby is getting this type of formula no other dietary iron is necessary. Most dry baby cereals are enriched with a form of iron that is easy for a baby's body to absorb. The prepared strained cereals differ in the amount of iron fortification and the form in which the iron is added. Certain cereal preparations contain no added iron; others contain iron in a chemical form that is less well absorbed into the bloodstream than the iron found in dry cereals. As discussed later in the chapter, new types of iron are now being tried for the fortification of "wet" cereals.

Human milk and cow's milk are not good sources of iron. Breast-fed babies are often given supplemental iron in the form of vitamin-mineral drops and/or are fed an iron-enriched baby cereal.

Baby food, formula, or supplements, along with the baby's own iron stores, provide most babies with sufficient iron during the first 6 months of life. During the second half of the first year and beyond, the baby's iron intake can drop drastically, as illustrated in the following cases:

1. The baby is switched from iron-fortified formula to cow's milk, and a reliable source of iron is thus eliminated.

2. The mother stops using a vitamin-mineral supplement because it is expensive, the baby is eating a variety of foods now, and the front of all his shirts are discolored from vitamin-mineral drool.

3. The baby is fed the family cereal because it is less expensive than baby cereal. Unless the cereal contains supplemental iron, a food source of iron is dropped from the baby's diet.

4. Although the baby is supposedly eating a variety of foods, he actually manages to subsist on two Cheerios, three banana slices, and one piece of hot dog each day. He is not hungry because he still drinks almost a quart of milk a day.

One or more of the above conditions can result in a sharp drop in dietary iron at a time when the iron stores with which the baby was born are becoming depleted. The only way to be sure the baby receives enough iron is to continue feeding him iron-fortified cereal (even though it costs slightly more than adult cereals) or give him an iron supplement. If the baby eats only limited quantities of a few foods throughout the second year of life, his dietary iron may continue to be insufficient. Keeping a list of everything the baby eats for a week before a routine checkup can help the pediatrician determine if iron or other nutrients are missing from the baby's diet. (It is important to include all foods eaten during the day, not just those served at mealtimes.)

Other Minerals

Although several other minerals should be supplied in the baby's diet, the precise requirement for many of them has not been established. Because deficiencies in these minerals are rare during infancy and early childhood, we can assume that milk fulfills the baby's need for them. The amount of these minerals added to commercial formula is based on their levels in human milk. A diet severely limited in variety and quantity for a prolonged period can of course cause deficiencies of these minerals, but such a diet would probably also be deficient in other vitamins and minerals for which the requirements are known. Therefore it has been difficult to distinguish specific signs of trace mineral malnutrition. However, new information about the requirements for, and functions of, these nutrients is accumulating rapidly. For example, zinc deficiency was recently found to be associated with a decreased ability to distinguish among tastes.

Fluoride is often added to vitamin and mineral supplements for babies because it helps to form decay-resistant teeth. It combines with a substance in tooth enamel to make fluorapatite, a compound not easily broken down by the acid produced by bacteria in the mouth. Because milk does not contain enough fluoride for optimal tooth formation during infancy, many pediatricians recommend fluoride supplements in the form of drops or, later on, chewable tablets. Fluoridated water is probably the best source of this mineral when teeth are forming because the body uses the mineral most effectively when it is consumed several times during the day.

A young baby is rarely given water more than once or twice a day. If he is fed a commercial infant formula diluted with tap water, he will consume considerable amounts of this mineral when he eats. Breast-fed infants do not have this alternative. Since most young children prefer to drink fluids other than water when they are thirsty, one way of increasing their intake of fluoridated water is to use powdered milk or frozen juices that must be reconstituted with tap water. Because this mineral is so important during the formation of teeth, parents might want to ensure that only water or beverages reconstituted with fluoridated water are available to their children during most of the day.

FEEDING PRACTICES

Feeding the baby can be divided into two phases: milk and solid food. This section discusses methods of feeding milk to the baby, the nutritional requirements of the nursing mother, the nutritional quality of commercial baby food, the increasing use of baby foods, and finally how attitudes toward food can be developed by early feeding practices.

Milk

Most babies are either breast-fed or fed a commercial formula that resembles, to a great extent, the composition of human milk (4). Despite the intensity and quantity of arguments used to convince a mother-to-be to breast-feed, no compelling evidence exists that human milk is significantly better *nutritionally* than formula. In fact, the vitamin D and iron fortification of formula makes it a better source of these nutrients than human milk. The other nutrients needed by the baby, however, are supplied in the necessary quantities in milk from a well-nourished mother, and human milk remains the most "natural" food a human being can receive.

The fat content and to a lesser degree the amounts of protein and amino acids in human milk vary considerably among women and even within the same woman from one nursing to another. Commercial formula does not change; its composition is based on the average amounts of specific nutrients in human milk, as determined by analyzing milk from thousands of women. The daily variations in the composition of human milk and the uniqueness of each nursing mother's milk may be as much a part of the special relationship a mother has with her baby as the way the infant is held or smiled at during a feeding.

Physicians now believe that human milk gives the baby some protection against organisms that can cause infections of the intestinal tract. Antibodies, proteins that destroy bacteria and viruses, are found in colostrum (fluid secreted from the breasts after the baby is born but before milk is produced) and to a lesser extent in milk itself. In addition, milk contains other substances that either prevent the growth of certain disease-causing microorganisms in the intestine or destroy them. This protective quality of milk is most useful for a baby raised in a home where lack of money and facilities makes sterilizing bottles and refrigerating formula impossible.

Breast milk therefore can be considered the optimal food for the infant; it is custom-made for the baby and, with vitamin D and iron supplements, meets all his nutritional needs up to the sixth month of life. Breast-feeding prevents bacterial contamination, protects against intestinal diseases, and eliminates the danger of overfeeding the baby.

The bottle-fed baby is vulnerable to certain hazards: the formula can become contaminated (although this risk is minimal under most circumstances in the United States); the baby can be overfed; and the concentration of the formula can be altered either by reducing or increasing the amount of water added. Babies are sometimes fed formulas containing less water than specified in order to "fill them up" for a longer period. This practice can be dangerous because the infant's body is unable to handle the increased amounts of protein and minerals found in a concentrated formula. Conversely, a formula may be diluted with excess water to make it last longer. (This practice sometimes occurs also when the family cannot afford to buy enough formula for the baby.) Young babies cannot drink enough of a watered formula to obtain the calories and nutrients they need, and this practice may result in a retarded growth rate.

Formula-fed babies might be switched to cow's milk earlier than breast-fed babies to eliminate the cost of formula from the family's food budget (cow's milk is much cheaper, especially if it is reconstituted from an evaporated or dried preparation). Unless the mother is advised to add supplemental iron to the baby's diet or uses an iron-fortified baby cereal, the child's consumption of cow's milk instead of formula can cause a sudden decrease in his iron intake. (Breast-feeding mothers are usually instructed about dietary sources of iron when the baby is quite yound since human milk contains less iron than iron-fortified formula.) Cow's milk contains more butterfat than does formula, and an infant's intestines cannot absorb it entirely. Fat eliminated in the feces represents calories lost to the infant and, if the switch to cow's milk is made at a time when the infant is receiving most of his calories from formula, he may be deprived of calories needed for growth. Pediatricians recommend waiting until the baby eats about one and a half to two jars of baby food a day before switching him from formula to cow's milk.

The bottle-fed child is also vulnerable to tooth decay caused by the "nursing bottle syndrome" mentioned earlier in the chapter. This is a hazard from which the breast-fed baby is immune.

Lest the reader think that breast-feeding is without difficulties, the following 1975 news item illustrates one of the hazards a nursing mother may encounter (8):

"Topless Swimmer" A Nursing Mother

> Someone telephoned a complaint to police at 2:35 p.m. on Saturday, saying there was a woman in topless attire on the Great Harbors shorefront. Responding to the alarm of public nudity, the police found a mother nursing her baby. They took no action.

Feeding the Nursing Mother

At first, the nursing mother produces about a quart of milk a day (700 to 900 milliliters), and as the baby grows older the volume can increase. Since this amount of milk contains a considerable quantity of nutrients—protein, calcium, zinc, lactose, fat, and other vitamins and minerals plus water—the lactating woman must use either her own stores of nutrients or those in her food for the milk she produces. The energy necessary for making milk is provided either by fat stores accumulated during pregnancy or by dietary calories. Not surprisingly, physicians usually expect nursing mothers to eat according to a list of required nutrients. For the most part, the quantities and kinds of foods needed during lactation are similar to those required during pregnancy; however, the amount of milk required increases during lactation. Tables 2 and 3 present nutrient requirements and the number of servings of various foods necessary to meet these requirements.

Theoretically, the pregnant or nursing mother would be a paragon of nutritional virtue if she faithfully consumed dark green leafy vegetables, milk, citrus fruits, and other worthwhile foods. In reality, many breast-feeding mothers, like their bottle-feeding counterparts, worry more about the differences in vitamin C content in strained applesauce and bananas than about their own food habits. Recently I asked some breast-feeding mothers to write down everything they ate on a given day when their babies were 4 to 6 weeks old in the hope of using their food choices as examples of what nursing mothers should be eating. Instead, the absence of adequate amounts of milk, vegetables, and in some cases protein and citrus fruits made me worry about their own nutritional status.

The demands made on the mother of a very young baby practically ensure that the nutritional demands of her own body are met last. She is more likely to be counting the number of clean diapers than thinking about the number of servings of turnip greens or whole wheat bread she is expected to eat. Her food choices may

TABLE 2. *Recommended Daily Dietary Allowances during lactation*

Nutrient[a]	Requirement
Energy (Kcal)	2,500
Protein (grams)	66
Vitamin A (IU)	6,000
Vitamin D (IU)	400
Vitamin E (IU)	15
Vitamin C (mg)	105
Folic acid (Folacin) (μg)[b]	600
Niacin (mg)	17
Riboflavin (mg)	1.7
Thiamin (mg)	1.3
Vitamin B_6 (mg)	2.5
Vitamin B_{12} (μg)	4.0
Calcium (mg)	1,200
Phosphorus (mg)	1,200
Iodine (μg)	150
Iron (mg)[b]	18
Magnesium (mg)	450
Zinc (mg)	25

From ref. 15.
Kcal = kilocalories. See Table 1 for other abbreviations.

[a]The amount of each nutrient is based on the requirements of a reference woman who is between the ages of 23 and 50 and weighs 128 pounds.

[b]Dietary supplements may be necessary to provide the recommended amounts of iron and folic acid, especially iron.

TABLE 3. *Servings and types of foods needed to meet Recommended Daily Dietary Allowances for lactating women*

Type of food	Examples	No. of servings
Protein (animal and vegetable)[a]	All	4
Milk and milk products	Milk, cottage cheese, yogurt	5
Grain products	Bread, pasta, rice, cereal, tortillas	3
Vitamin-C-rich fruits and vegetables	Citrus fruits, tomatoes, green peppers, cabbage, strawberries	1
Leafy green vegetables	Cabbage, broccoli, kale, spinach, asparagus, chicory, escarole, watercress	2
Other vegetables and fruits	Carrots, corn, celery, lettuce, beets, potatoes, apples, pears, bananas, sweet potatoes, squash, eggplant, mushrooms, peas	1

From ref. 16.

[a]Vegetable protein combinations should contain complementary essential amino acids; see Chapters 2 and 5.

revert to prepregnancy patterns—foods the family eats, especially items that can be cooked and served quickly.

However, the nutritional demands on the mother continue as long as she nurses; and if she nurses for 3 to 4 months without replenishing her nutrient stores through her diet, she may leave this period of lactation with depleted stores of nutrients and possibly diminished nutritional health. In addition, the vitamin and mineral content of the milk depends on the supply of these nutrients in the mother's blood. Although most mothers manage to maintain normal levels of vitamins and minerals in their milk, a woman whose diet entirely lacks certain vitamins or minerals can produce milk with lower than normal levels of these nutrients.

Prenatal nutrition counseling often includes advice about what the mother should eat during the lactation period. The baby's pediatrician should ask the mother about her eating habits as well as those of her baby and, if necessary, suggest ways of improving her diet. Since the breast-feeding mother provides the major source of food for her child, the pediatrician can legitimately be concerned about her nutritional status. Although it may be heresy to say this, a woman should *not* consider breast-feeding if the associated nutritional demands conflict with her anticipated life style. A woman who drinks milk through clenched teeth during pregnancy and detests cheese, cottage cheese, and yogurt may contemplate 2 or 3 more months of that "white stuff" with horror; and the lady who plans on starving herself into a postnatal bikini is more apt to eliminate than to add foods to her diet, even though she is told to do so in order to breast-feed well.

The La Leche League[12] is a valuable source of nutritional as well as general

[12]For more information, contact the La Leche League International, 96916 Minneapolis Ave., Franklin Park, Illinois 60131.

information about breast-feeding. This organization has local chapters, and the members provide personal support and suggestions to the novice nursing mother.

Weaning Foods

Weaning is defined as the process of "accustoming the child to food other than mother's milk" (9). Until early in this century, this "process" was initiated only after the baby had several teeth (usually at 8 to 12 months of age), and then only small amounts of high-carbohydrate mush were fed. This practice contrasts with the current trend of weaning the infant almost immediately after birth; some pediatricians recommend feeding baby food to the infant as early as 1 week of age.

The first weaning foods are usually cereals, followed by strained fruits and juices. If the baby accepts these foods (usually determined by the bib test—if more food is on the bib than in the baby—the mother should wait before introducing more foods), a colorful array of strained vegetables (red beets, green beans, yellow squash, and carrots) and strained meats, eggs, and combination dinners are then offered. The variety of baby foods available today must be seen to be believed. The baby food section of a supermarket resembles a miniature, strained version of the supermarket itself. Eggs and bacon, hot dog dinners, chicken and noodle casseroles, Dutch apple desert, and blueberry buckle are among the foods displayed to tempt the mother, if not the infant.

Experts on infant nutrition contend that formula or human milk plus the appropriate vitamin and mineral supplements satisfies the infant's nutritional needs up to the sixth month. Many such pediatricians advise delaying the introduction of baby food until that age, but few mothers do. Recent surveys of infant feeding practices in this country and in England indicated that 90% of all babies are receiving some type of weaning food by 3 months of age or earlier (10–12). Since many mothers associate the ability of their offspring to swallow applesauce with intellectual development, it is unlikely that this trend will soon change.

Two problems may result from premature introduction of baby foods. Cereals and strained fruits, the foods most commonly fed to the young infant, are high in carbohydrate and low in protein. Filling a baby with these foods may cause him to drink less milk and thus reduce his protein consumption. When he is old enough to eat a variety of high-protein baby foods (meat, cheese, eggs) a decrease in his consumption of milk will not affect his total protein intake.

The other problem concerns the baby who does not drink less milk when fed baby food. If he eats a jar of strained bananas or chocolate pudding and then drinks the same amount of milk he would have had without the serving of baby food, he is probably consuming too many calories. Such babies may be candidates for the diaper branch of Weight Watchers and may develop a lifelong weight problem. Although not all fat babies become fat adults, several studies (13,14) have pointed to a relationship between fat young (6 months or younger) infants

TABLE 4. *Content of three minerals in oatmeal*

Form of oatmeal (⅓ cup)	Iron (mg)	Calcium (mg)	Phosphorus (mg)
Dry infant variety	14.2	94	99
Strained, with fruit	1.7	27	33
Rolled oats	1.3	15	115

and obese adults. Baby food is useful and necessary when milk can no longer meet the caloric or nutrient needs of the infant. Before that time, however, its nutritional utility is questionable.[13]

Baby foods differ in nutrient content, and the following section notes the major nutritional characteristics of various types of food. These products change continually, however, so reading labels may be necessary for updating nutritional information.

Cereals

Baby cereal comes in two forms: dry and strained. Owing to differences in mineral fortification, their nutritional values differ significantly. Table 4 compares the calcium, phosphorus, and iron content of three forms of oatmeal: dry infant oatmeal, a strained baby food oatmeal containing applesauce and bananas, and adult oatmeal (4).

The difference in iron content among the three types of cereal is considerable and supports the advice of many pediatricians that a baby should be fed iron-fortified dry baby cereal even when old enough to eat the family variety. [A strained cereal-fruit preparation fortified with iron appeared recently in the supermarkets. The chemical form of iron (ferrous sulfate) used in the fortification is similar to that used to fortify baby formulas and is easily absorbed by the baby's body.]

Fruit Juices

All baby fruit juices are fortified with 50 milligrams of ascorbic acid (vitamin C), which is more than twice the daily vitamin C requirement for infants (20 milligrams). Among the "adult" juices a baby might find palatable (apple, grape, and orange), only orange juice contains similar amounts of vitamin C (60 milligrams) in the quantity a baby is able to drink (about 4 fluid ounces). Therefore, unless the adult form of grape or apple juice is fortified with ascorbic acid, the infant variety should be used to add vitamin C to the baby's diet.

---

[13]The concern over infant obesity and subsequent adult obesity has led some mothers to restrict the caloric intake of their infants. This practice is even more dangerous than overfeeding since the nutrient intake also may be restricted. The baby should be the final judge of how much to eat; breast-fed babies manage to eat the right amount without maternal intervention.

Vegetables and Fruits

The labels on jars of strained fruits and vegetables indicate if the item contains added sugar and cornstarch. Since these ingredients do not add to the nutritive value of the food, it is not necessary to feed them to the baby. A careful selection of brands provides these foods in a filler-free form. Careful label reading is important, and a magnifying glass can help since the print is very small. Caution: Do not attempt to analyze labels when accompanied to the market by a small infant and the week's shopping list. The best time to investigate the contents of commercial baby foods is the week before the baby is born, when the kitchen is not only clean but also contains two impatient grandmothers.

Desserts and Puddings

Most desserts are inadequate sources of nutrients and, like adult desserts, should be regarded as items of culinary pleasure rather than of nutritional benefit. Milk-based desserts (e.g., butterscotch or cherry-vanilla pudding) are good sources of riboflavin and vitamin A, but of course so is milk. The fruit and pastry desserts (Dutch apple dessert, blueberry buckle, peach cobbler) provide primarily calories.

Strained Meats and Meat Dinners

The protein content of strained meat and meat dinners varies considerably, and these items should be selected with care. These foods, along with egg and meat combination dinners, are usually the main course and, as such, represent the protein component of the baby's meal. The amount of protein fed to a baby during a given meal should be equivalent to the amount he would receive in milk during a feeding period, since his milk consumption will decrease considerably as he becomes used to solid foods.

Strained meat preparations (e.g., beef, veal, or liver) contain the most protein; dinners of meat and extraneous bits of vegetables or noodles contain less protein but are still a good source of this nutrient. Vegetable and meat combination dinners contain the least protein. In Table 5 the protein content of three baby foods shows this relationship (4).

TABLE 5. *Protein-calorie relationships in three baby foods*

Baby food (1 jar)	Protein per gram	% Caloric content
Strained beef (99 grams or 3.5 oz)	13.4	60
High-meat beef dinner with vegetables (128 grams or 4.5 oz)	7.8	30
Vegetable and beef combination dinner (128 grams or 4.5 oz)	2.5	15

Baby Food: Homemade or Commercial?

Grinding and blending baby food at home is an increasingly popular trend, much to the bewilderment of many grandmothers who had no choice but to wrestle with food mills, strainers, and mortar and pestle each time the baby was fed solid food. To these grandmothers and those before them, commercial baby food symbolized the end of tedious preparations and, perhaps just as important, the availability of reliable products prepared under standardized and sterile conditions. Mothers defend their return to homemade baby foods by claiming that their product is cleaner, less expensive, and more nutritious. Let us briefly consider their arguments to establish if homemade baby food is indeed better for the baby than the store-bought variety.

Safety

Bacterial contamination of commercial baby food is virtually unknown because sterilization procedures are highly developed and scrupulously followed. Indeed homemade baby food is more vulnerable to bacterial contamination, especially in warm weather, and the mother must be careful to follow proper cooking and refrigeration procedures. On the other hand, contamination by rodent and insect particles has been found in commercial baby foods and acknowledged by spokesmen for baby food companies. Although any contamination of this type is unacceptable to a mother and justifiably criticized, a curious, crawling baby exploring the world through his mouth will ingest more of these "particles" in an afternoon than in a year or more of eating commercial baby food.

Nutrition

The preparation of commercial baby food requires the addition of considerably more water than would be added to the same food prepared at home. Consequently the nutrient content is diluted. For example, 1 teaspoon of homemade chicken and noodle dinner contains more carbohydrate, protein, fat, vitamins, minerals, and calories than the commercial preparation. As mentioned earlier, commercial baby foods often contain sodium and, depending on the type of food, sugar and food starch. The vitamin and mineral content of commercial baby foods, however, is relatively constant. Although nutrients are lost during processing, standardized methods of preparation are used to minimize variations among different batches of food. Nutrient loss also occurs in homemade preparations, and the absence of a standard method of cooking from one kitchen to another can cause enormous variations in the mineral and vitamin content of homemade baby foods. Therefore the method of preparation should reduce nutrient loss, otherwise the vitamin and mineral content of baby food made at home may be actually less than that found in a similar commercial product, even though the ingredients are not diluted with water.

Cost

If homemade baby food is prepared from the same ingredients as the family meals, it probably costs less than a commercial product; but if small amounts of produce or meat must be bought especially for baby food, commercial preparations are cheaper.

Using both homemade and commercial baby food can cause some confusion in estimating the amount of food to feed the baby. Since homemade baby food is nutritionally and calorically denser than commercial baby food, a mother must not expect her baby to consume as much of it as of the store-bought variety. Doing so may lead to overfeeding.

The choice of baby food depends more on personal considerations than nutritional, economic, or safety factors. No clear-cut advantage of one type over the other now exists; however, the choice should bring maternal satisfaction, and this is as good a basis as any for making the decision.

Feeding and Eating Patterns

Feeding a baby is more than putting food in his mouth. The feeding process conveys attitudes and associations about food that eventually become part of the baby's personal style of eating as an adult. Developing an individual eating style continues into adulthood; however, many basic feelings about eating are initiated early in life, and these may be the most resistant to change later on. Foods and flavors become linked with physical and emotional events, and act as vaguely remembered cues that direct food choices throughout life. For example, for centuries parents have used sweet-tasting foods to comfort a child. During the eighteenth century giving a baby a piece of rag dipped in honey had the same effect as distracting a crying, whining child with ice cream or a cookie today: a cessation of noise and a momentary forgetting of the reason for the noise. When this feeding event is repeated often enough, an association is formed between the sweet taste on the tongue and the relief of discomfort. As an adult, this individual may almost unconsciously eat a sweet food during a stressful or anxious period because of the learned expectations that the sweet taste will make him "feel better."

Should a parent attempt to avoid the development of this "sweet-comfort" relationship by relieving the infant's distress with a taste of pickle juice or an anchovy, he will fail. The adult enjoyment of salty or sour foods is absent in the young infant, and his response will probably be an increase in distress. Theoretically, the parent should avoid the entire association between food and comfort by using a nonfood response to the baby's nonhunger needs.

Overfeeding is another hazard. The bottle-fed baby is often confronted with it almost immediately. Draining the bottle is an event that produces great joy in an inexperienced mother, and the baby, coaxed into finishing the final ounce, may learn that a too-full stomach is a small price to pay for the smiles and compliments accompanying this feat. Conversely, stern expressions, such as, "the next time, you can cry longer for your bottle," are sometimes used when the baby simply plays with the nipple rather than finishing his milk. The breast-fed baby escapes this dilemma, because the nursing mother has no way of knowing, accurately, the amount of milk her baby has consumed. Obesity among bottle-fed babies is thought to be due in part to the mother's attempt to determine how much milk the baby should consume. Once the breast-fed baby is given supplemental bottle feedings, he is also vulnerable to being overfed. This danger also accompanies the feeding of baby food; emptying the dish or jar of baby food are goals set by the mother, which may be incompatible with the caloric or nutrient needs of the baby. If eating everything represents eating too much, then this overfeeding may produce not only a fat baby but also an adult who feels compelled to "clean the plate" regardless of the amount on it, and who, by doing so, may continue to overeat.

As mentioned earlier, some mothers have the opposite attitude toward the amount of food their babies eat. Their motto is, "the less the better." Aside from the nutritional hazards inherent in such an attitude, these children may develop feelings of anxiety about food, especially if they are always a little hungry.

Babies are able to regulate their food intake by the time they are about 6 weeks old; and if they are breast-fed, or bottle-fed without being coaxed to increase their consumption, they manage to eat enough to meet their nutrient needs for maintenance and growth. Allowing a baby to develop a sense of hunger and to discover how much food is needed to satisfy it will help him to recognize the cues he needs to regulate his body weight as he grows older.

Finally, development of a personal eating style is influenced by the factors that determine how the family eats. Ethnic or religious customs and geographic, economic, and cultural factors participate in having the young baby become accustomed to foods and attitudes about food that characterize his particular family.

REFERENCES

1. Wood, A. (1968): The history of artificial feeding of infants. In: *Lydia J. Roberts Award Essays.* American Dietetic Association, Chicago.
2. Bracken, F. (1968): Infant feeding in the American colonies. In: *Lydia J. Roberts Award Essays.* American Dietetic Association, Chicago.
3. Church, C., and Church, H. (1975): *Food Values of Portions Commonly Used,* 12th ed. Lippincott, Philadelphia.
4. Fomon, S. (1974): *Infant Nutrition,* 2nd ed. Saunders, Philadelphia.
5. Underwood, B., Hepner, R., and Hadjea, A. (1970): Protein, lipid and fatty acids of human milk from Pakistani women during prolonged periods of lactation. *Am. J. Clin. Nutr.* 23:400–407.
6. Gunasekara, D.B., and Wijesinha, G.S. (1956): Composition of breast milk of some Ceylonese mothers with a note on the age of weaning in Ceylon. *Ceylon J. Med. Sci.,* 9:23–29.
7. Jacobs, H., Smutz, E., and DuBose, C.(1976):Taste preference. In: *Taste and Development,The Genesis of Sweet Preference,* edited by J. Weiffenbach. Government Printing Office, Washington, D.C.
8. *Falmouth Enterprise.* Falmouth, Mass., July 9, 1975.
9. *Oxford English Dictionary.* Oxford University Press, New York, 1933.
10. Fomon, S. (1975): What are infants fed in the United States. *Pediatrics,* 56:350–354.

11. Taitz, L.S. (1971): Infantile overnutrition among artificially fed infants in Sheffield region. *Br. Med. J.,* 1:315–321.
12. Shukla, A., Forsyth, H.A., Anderson, C., and Marwah, S.M. (1972): Infantile overnutrition in the first year of life. *Br. Med. J.,* 2:507–515.
13. Charney, E., Chamblee, H., Goodman, R.N., McBridge, M., Lyon, B., and Pratt, R. (1976): Childhood antecedents of adult obesity. *N. Engl. J. Med.,* 295:6–9.
14. Eid, E.E. (1970): Follow-up study of physical growth of children who had excessive weight gain in the first six months of life. *Br. Med. J.,* 2:74.
15. National Academy of Sciences (1979): *Recommended Dietary Allowances,* 9th ed. National Academy of Sciences, Washington, D.C. *(in press).*
16. Cunningham, G., editor (1975): *Nutrition During Lactation.* California Department of Health, Sacramento.

7 THE INDEPENDENT EATER: Nutrition During Childhood and Adolescence

Eating during childhood and adolescence has two effects. It supplies the nutrients needed for physical growth and development, and it provides many of the associations with food that influence the child's personal eating style as an adult.

The nutritional quality of the diet during these years is critically important because physical growth is completed by the end of adolescence. (All subsequent growth takes place from side to side.) This chapter discusses the specific nutrient needs of childhood and adolescence and, in addition, indicates which foods containing these nutrients are *likely to be eaten.*

Unfortunately, the chapter does not provide a failproof way for getting a child or teenager to eat nutritious foods. As one of the sections points out, there seems to be a critical period during these years when it may be possible to program a child to eat only nutritious foods. This period lasts about 6 weeks, after the child leaves the highchair and before he is hypnotized by Saturday morning television shows. This period should be watched for carefully because, if missed, the child's willingness to eat foods promoted by the mother begins to fade. We should heed the old adage—found in an abandoned freezer filled with boxes of frozen spinach, broccoli, carrots, corn, kale, beets, and peas—"you can't feed an old child new vegetables." If this period is missed, however, you still may be able to influence a child to make nutritious food choices some of the time, or at least teach him to approach vegetables with less revulsion than adults have for eating eels.

Associations with food made during childhood continue to affect eating throughout adult life. This chapter also focuses on the child's eating environment in order to understand these factors and their influence on the nutritional quality of the diet. We are all familiar with these associations. Memories of steak on birthdays, egg salad sandwiches during second grade, and a bowl of corn chowder immediately before we got sick continue to determine whether we eat these foods as adults. By the time childhood and adolescence are over, the individual usually can categorize foods as preferred, neutral, or disliked; and he has a well-established pattern set for the foods he eats and the appropriate time and place to eat them. (We all learn at some point during childhood that salami and sauerkraut are not acceptable breakfast foods and that hot dogs are inappropriate for Thanksgiving dinner.) These patterns of food choice have a direct influence on the nutritional quality of the diet, and if the patterns are incompatible with nutrient needs they may result in chronic nutritional inadequacies or excesses (e.g., avoidance of vegetables containing needed vitamins and minerals, or excessive intake of calories or high-fat foods). It is therefore critically important to reinforce nutritionally sound food associations during childhood and adolescence; this chapter describes factors that may enhance or hinder this objective.

A LOOK AT THE PAST

Today children may eat poorly, but it is often by choice. In the past, ignorance, lack of money, and limited availability of many foods caused children to grow up ill-fed and often marked by rickets, a common nutrient deficiency disease. A record of what children were once fed is found in the diet sheets and bills of English orphanages and boarding schools. During the eighteenth century, for example, children were rarely given vegetables and fruits, except potatoes, and often one food (e.g., bread) was considered sufficient for a meal. The November 1747 diet sheet from the Foundling Hospital (1) gives a typical menu. Breakfast was broth, gruel, or milk porridge; dinner was roast or boiled meat, puddings or potato; and supper was bread, milk and bread, or bread and cheese. Interestingly, the diet for the staff included considerably more meat plus a variety of vegetables, e.g., turnips, greens, carrots, "roots" (parsnips and squash), and lentils. The children's diet was clearly deficient in vitamins; that of the adults was not. Boarding schools such as Christ' Hospital provided similarly inadequate fare. This led a physician during the late eighteenth century to comment that the boys were "seldom glutted with quantity...and farinaceous cereal foods are generally esteemed the best or *rather the cheapest* [author's italics] for them" (1).

Scurvy was common in boarding schools, and eventually potatoes were added to the diet because it was observed that they decreased the frequency of this disease. (Recognition that potatoes contain vitamin C did not come for two more centuries.) Vegetables and fruits continued to be ignored until the end of the nineteenth century; and scurvey, rickets, and nutritional anemias were common among the young.

Until the middle of the nineteenth century, the amount of food needed to meet the energy requirements of both adults and children was unknown, and usually the food given to adults in poorhouses and prisons was calorically insufficient. (There also were, no doubt, social reasons for keeping these people half-starved.) Even after the caloric requirements of the adult were known, however, no one realized that children, because they are growing, need more calories in relation to their weight than adults. Children in institutions and schools continued to be fed inadequate amounts of food. This is described most poignantly by Charles Dickens in *Nicholas Nickleby* (2) when he talks about the "pale and haggard faces," and "boys of stunted growth, and others whose long meagre legs would hardly bear their stooping bodies."

By the early twentieth century, nutritional research began to define the nutrient needs of children, and feeding practices improved slowly. Unfortunately, during this time children's diets were often poor for another reason, lack of money. The large numbers of poorly paid immigrants in this country, unemployment in Europe and the United States, and the high cost of food in the cities (compared with the cheapness of food grown by the back door) caused the quantity and variety of foods children ate to remain inadequate.

By 1935 some states in the United States provided free lunches for poor children; however, it was not until 1946 that the National School Lunch Act provided all children with a lunchtime meal. The meal was designed to contain one-third of the daily nutrient requirements for children and made a significant difference in the nutrient intake of otherwise poorly fed children. (More recently, the Child Nutrition Act of 1966 authorized a school breakfast program in schools with a high enrollment of the needy.) The increased size of children during the second half of this century compared to earlier generations reflects the improvement in their diets.

> Nutrition alone is not responsible for the increased stature of today's children; the eradication of many childhood diseases through immunization (polio, diphtheria, measles, mumps) and the decrease in the severity of many others through the use of antibiotics (strep throats rarely progress to scarlet fever these days) has had a pronounced influence.
>
> Children do not grow when they are sick; if sickness is infrequent and brief, the loss of growth time is almost imperceptible. In the past (and also currently in developing countries) children were sick often and for prolonged periods of time. Bacterial infections of the ears and throat were common and were often accompanied by a loss of appetite and/or restricted diet. (Chicken soup, tea, and toast are fine for a sick child but are limited nutritionally.) Therefore children recovered from a sickness in a somewhat depleted nutritional state; and if another illness occurred soon after, the disease and lack of nutrients combined to slow the growth rate.

There are still areas in the United States today where children with deficiencies of iron, vitamin A, thiamin, and riboflavin are not uncommon. Recently a survey published by HEW showed that the growth rate was slower than normal among children from economically depressed parts of the country (3).

Poor food choices also affect the nutritional adequacy of the diet, and children who eat a junk food-based diet can be found all over the country. Their food intake often resembles that of the children in the eighteenth century Foundling Hospital in terms of its vegetable and fruit content. Eating many meals away from home, susceptibility to advertising, the nutritional "illiteracy" of many mothers, and peer pressure to eat like everyone else conspire to prevent children from obtaining their needed nutrients.

NUTRIENT NEEDS OF CHILDHOOD AND ADOLESCENCE

The nutrient needs of children and adolescents are listed in Table 1. The amounts shown are deceptive in that they are so much smaller than the amounts listed for adults (Chapter 2). They seem to indicate that a child really could subsist on a diet of chocolate cupcakes, a slice of cheese, potato chips, and milk. Because the nutrient needs of the child and adolescent are *related to their weight,* however, their needs are proportionately far greater than adult requirements. Growth uses up the additional nutrients and calories for the formation of new tissue. The graph

TABLE 1. Recommended Daily Dietary Allowances[a] for children and adolescents

Nutrient	Requirements for children ages 1–10			Requirements for preteens and teenagers ages 11–18			
	1–3	4–6	7–10	11–14 Male	11–14 Female	15–18 Male	15–18 Female
Energy (calories)	1,300	1,800	2,400	2,800	2,400	3,000	2,100
Protein	23	30	36	44	44	54	48
Vitamin A							
RE	400	500	700	1,000	800	1,000	800
IU	2,000	2,500	3,300	5,000	4,000	5,000	4,000
Vitamin D (IU)	400	400	400	400	400	400	400
Vitamin E (IU)	7	9	10	12	12	15	12
Ascorbic acid (mg)	65	65	65	70	70	70	70
Folacin (µg)	100	200	300	400	400	400	400
Niacin (mg)	9	12	16	18	16	20	14
Riboflavin (mg)	0.8	1.1	1.2	1.5	1.3	1.8	1.4
Thiamin (mg)	0.7	0.9	1.2	1.4	1.2	1.5	1.1
Vitamin B_{12} (µg)	1.0	1.5	2.0	3.0	3.0	3.0	3.0
Vitamin B_6 (mg)	0.6	0.9	1.2	1.6	1.6	2.0	2.0
Calcium (mg)	800	800	800	1,200	1,200	1,200	1,200
Phosphorus (mg)	800	800	800	1,200	1,200	1,200	800
Iodine (µg)	60	80	110	130	115	150	115
Iron (mg)	15	10	10	18	18	18	18
Magnesium (mg)	150	200	250	350	300	400	300
Zinc (mg)	10	10	10	15	15	15	15

RE = retinal equivalents. IU = international units; mg = milligrams; µg = micrograms.

[a]From Food and Nutrition Board, National Academy of Sciences-National Research Council, 1979.

in Fig. 1 shows the speed with which boys and girls grow from year to year. It is evident that children grow all the time, although not always at the same rate.

Infants grow progressively less rapidly from birth on (a baby may double its birth weight by 3 months of age, going, for example, from 7 to 14 pounds. However, if he continued to grow at the same rate, he would weigh 152 pounds at 1 year. In general, the growth of children slows down continually until they are 9 to 10 (girls) or 12.5 to 13 (boys) years of age. At this age, which coincides with the onset of puberty, the rate of growth speeds up. A boy can grow as fast at age 13 to 14 as he last did when he was 2 years old. (Parents of young infants and teenagers are continually amazed at the rapid changes in size occurring almost before their eyes. Babies outgrow their baby gifts before they can be worn and teenagers outgrow their clothes before they are worn out.)

At some point between 6 months and 2 years of age, a child's rate of growth slows down dramatically (Fig. 1). Because the growth rate has decreased, appetite decreases too. The change, although normal, can upset parents who are not prepared for it.

A young mother who boasted of her son's gustatory feats was reduced to tears when, at 18 months, he suddenly rejected all the foods for which he once cried and insisted on eating only apple juice and cookies for 3 weeks. She was sure he was developing a bizarre eating disorder; actually, he was simply reflecting the appetite of his age group.

Along with a decrease in the quantity of food eaten, there is usually a decrease in the variety of foods the child accepts. This fickleness may persist during the entire preschool period. Often an addiction to one or two foods develops; the child lives on nothing else for months and then, without warning, refuses to eat another mouthful. And Mom is left with a year's supply of peanut butter and canned spaghetti her 3-year-old craved until yesterday.

Conversely, the amount and variety of acceptable foods may increase dramatically at adolescence: Charlie Brown, in a *Peanuts* cartoon, announces one day that he has "outgrown his lunch." Mother puts more in the lunch bag and the refrigerator and still cannot keep either the teenager or the refrigerator filled. Whether a child rejects food or is insatiable, these normal changes in eating habits can affect the adequacy of his nutrient intake.

Calories

Caloric requirements grow with the child. Adolescent boys have the highest absolute daily caloric requirements of anyone (3,000 kilocalories per day from 15 to 22 years of age). After growth ceases, caloric needs drop and the adult must proceed toward his waning years accompanied by waning caloric needs (and often by a waxing waist). If we look at caloric needs in relation to weight, however, the consumer of the most calories per pound is the infant from birth to 6 months of age. After that age, the absolute caloric requirement continues to increase, but the number of calories needed per pound decreases.

Charts are, at best, a rough estimate of the caloric needs of different age groups.

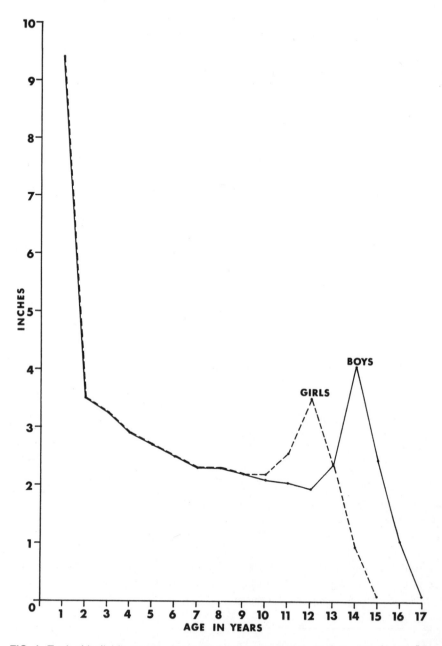

FIG. 1. Typical individual rate of growth for boys and girls. (Adapted from ref. 13.)

To begin with, they are based on the assumption that the child or teenager is a "typical" size and body frame, and that his growth rate is normal for a particular age group. A teenager who begins his growth spurt earlier or later than average may have caloric needs which differ from those in Table 1. Energy requirements of the child and teenager are based on two factors: in addition to the energy costs of growth (which are fairly standard for each age group); the basal metabolic energy needs and the energy consumed by physical activity.

> The basal metabolic rate indicates the energy needs of the body for its basic processes: breathing, producing hormones and enzymes, the work of muscles in maintaining posture and position, the beating of the heart, producing new cells, and many other functions. It is related to the total size of the individual, and so the basal metabolic needs of a child are less than those of an adult.

Physical activity is the most difficult to standardize with each age group, as activity levels vary widely among individuals—and even in the same individual from one season of the year to another. The following example illustrates this.

> One family has two school-age children (6 and 9). During the winter they are driven to school in the morning, walk home at 2:30, and spend the rest of the afternoon indoors, watching TV or playing, e.g., painting, clay sculpting, weaving. They usually go to bed around 8:00 or 8:30. During the late spring and summer they walk to school and back, then stay outside and play (running, climbing, or tumbling types of games); they eat supper and then go outside again. During summer vacation they go to sleep about a half-hour later than during the school year.
>
> The energy needs of these children must be different during the "outdoor" and the "indoor" months. If they are eating exactly the same all year round, they may be getting either an excess of calories during the winter or an inadequate amount during the summer. Ironically, children tend to eat more during the winter because they are indoors, near a refrigerator, and often eat as a diversion. During the warmer months children may drink more but often eat less because they fill up on fruit juice, water, or soda, and sometimes because they "can't be bothered" to stop their playing long enough to eat.

It is very difficult to monitor a child's caloric intake unless the child is studied in a clinical setting or the mother carries a log and records everything the child eats, outside as well as inside the home. Snacking begins at an extremely young age: The baby in the carriage is offered licks of an ice cream cone, and the toddler is given lollipops by the bank teller, cookies by the woman in the bakery, and anything at hand to distract him while his mother is conversing with a friend. Children sent to day-care centers at a young age probably eat well-controlled meals and snacks; however, unless the mother asks what and how much the child ate when she picks him up, she has no idea whether most or few of his caloric needs were satisfied during the day. The school-age child eats few of his meals or snacks under his mother's eye. He often grabs breakfast on the way out the door or gives it to the dog while his mother is finding his sneakers or writing a note for school; lunch is supposedly eaten at school (although the ratio of food eaten to that thrown or traded away has never been calculated). Snacks are often purchased either going to or returning from school (there is a candy shop near our local elementary school which does as brisk a business in candy bars at 8 a.m. as at 3 p.m.); if a friend has a filled cookie jar in the kitchen, snacking may be done in other homes during the afternoon. Caloric excesses or deficiencies caused by this peripatetic eating are eventually reflected by the weight gained at the end of 6 months or a year. An excess or insufficient weight gain may necessitate some scrutiny of the child's eating habits, not only to regulate his caloric intake but to make sure the calories he is consuming contain the nutrients he should be getting while he grows.

A mother's awareness of her child's nutritional needs can be complicated by the normal slowing of growth and consequent decrease in food intake, which occurs at about 1 year of age (Fig. 2). Since this is a natural occurrence, no mother should

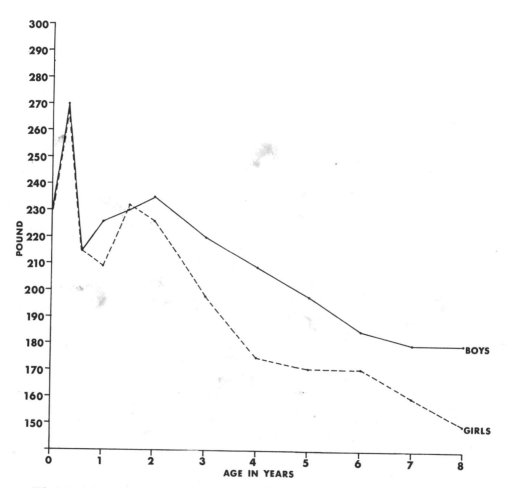

FIG. 2. Number of calories eaten per pound of body weight in children 0 to 8 years of age. (Information adapted from ref. 14.)

feel guilty or rejected because her child suddenly loses interest in food. However, if a child stops eating at mealtime and seems to be living "on air," it may be time to check out his snacking habits. A child can very nicely survive on milk, juice, cookies, ice cream cones, lollipops, and other snacks gathered in the course of the day's wanderings. Table 2 lists the food intake of a 2-year-old recorded several times over a 2-month period. When the record was first kept, it revealed that the boy ate most of his food in the form of snacks and juices. Two months later, after some suggestions were made to the mother about decreasing the availability of cookies and encouraging the child to eat adult food with the family, there was a decided improvement in the variety of foods he ate.

By keeping track of all the food eaten by the youngster for a day or so, a mother can learn whether any of it falls into the nutritious category (milk, fruits, vegetables, meat, breads, cereals, cheese, yogurt) or is comprised mainly of nonnutritious snack foods.

A food record chart that can be used to keep track of what and when a child eats is shown in Table 3. It is not necessary to record the amount of food eaten; however, if the child eats less than a crumb, teaspoon, fragment, sliver, or swallow of some food, it should not be recorded. Otherwise, the mother may overestimate what is actually eaten. When the child is old enough to talk and become aware of what he is eating, he can cooperate by telling his mother what he ate when she was not around (as at a day-care center). The chart is most useful for anticipating periods of the day when the child does most of his snacking. For example, if the youngster likes to eat at 3:00 in the afternoon, feeding him supper at that time will satisfy his hunger with nutritious foods. He can then have milk and a snack food in the early evening.

Finally, it should be noted that many children settle on a pattern of food intake rather early in childhood; they seem to follow a fairly constant caloric intake relative to their growth rate and size, and establish definite categories of acceptable or nonacceptable foods. Some children have rather small appetites, are satisfied quickly, and are simply unable to eat the quantities of food their mothers believe are necessary. Parents who use coercion or bribery to "convince" their offspring to clean their plates usually fail. Day-to-day warfare develops, which the child often wins by subterfuge. The dog or cat may become very fat, or the child may find clever hiding places for the food.

A prominent (thin) scientist recalls that he managed to defeat his mother's endeavors to make him eat by stuffing the extra food into a drawer in the kitchen table. The drawer contained silverware that was used only once a year, so when it was finally opened it contained, in addition to the silverware, a year's accumulation of very moldy food.

Children who lose these battles remember them bitterly. As adults, they are always ready to talk about how their mothers forced them to eat.

Protein

Protein requirements increase with age, reaching adult levels by late adolescence. Meat, fish, eggs, milk, and other dairy products are all good protein

TABLE 2. *Food intake of a 2-year-old boy*

Time	Food	Amount
	One day in February	
8:30 am	Water	3 oz
	Orange juice	3 oz
	Bread with margarine	1 slice
8:45	Ovaltine	4 oz
1:45 pm	Graham crackers	3
3:00	Ice cream and water	1 scoop ice cream
5:10	Macaroni and cheese	½ can
	Apple, peeled	1
	Milk	2 oz
	One week later	
8:00 am	Bread with margarine	1 slice
	Apple juice	3 oz
9:30	Graham cracker	1
10:30	Oatmeal cookie	1
	Lemonade	2 oz
	Apple juice	2 oz
11:45	Yogurt	4 oz
3:00 pm	Oatmeal cookies	2
	Chocolate chip cookie	1
5:15	Macaroni and cheese	¼ can
	Two months later	
8:00 am	Rice cereal	3 oz
	Milk	2 oz
11:45	Buttermilk pancakes with syrup	2½
	Cheese and crackers	½ oz cheese
		3 crackers
5:30 p.m.	Sirloin steak	3 oz
	Corn on the cob	½ cob
	Syrian bread	½ loaf (1 oz)
	Doughnut	½
	Milk	2 oz

The child took a vitamin and fluoride supplement each day containing the following vitamins: 1,500 IU vitamin A, 2 mg thiamin, 10 mg vitamin D, 2 mg riboflavin, 75 mg vitamin C. Ovaltine, which the child drank the first day his food intake was recorded, is fortified with several nutrients. One serving (¾ oz of ovaltine) contains the following concentration of nutrients, expressed as percent of the RDA for adults: protein 2%, vitamin A 45%, vitamin C 45%, thiamin 45%, riboflavin 45%, niacin 45%, calcium 8%, iron 15%, vitamin D 45%, vitamin B_6 45%, phosphorus 8%. The ovaltine is supposed to be mixed with 8 ounces of milk. Since the child drank only 4 ounces of milk, presumably he obtained only half the amount of the nutrients listed.

TABLE 3. *Record of child's daily food intake*

	Morning	Midday	Afternoon	Early evening
Fluids				
Water				
Milk				
Juice (apple, orange, cranberry, prune, grapefruit, pineapple)				
Fruit drink (powdered or canned)				
Soda				
Bread products				
Bread				
Muffins				
Pancakes				
Waffles				
Bagel				
Roll				
Toaster pastry				
Spaghetti				
Macaroni				
Other pastas				
Fruit				
Citrus				
Other				
Vegetables				
Potatoes				
Carrots				
Peas				
Salad				
Other				
Protein sources				
Beef				
Chicken				
Lamb				
Pork				
Tunafish				
Sardines				
Salmon				
Other fish				
Eggs				
Peanut butter				
Nuts				
Beans				
Bean curd				
Spreads				
Margarine, butter				
Cream cheese				
Jam, mashmallow fluff				
Snacks				
Dried fruits (raisins)				
Nuts, seeds				
Candy				
Cookies				
Crackers				
Other pastries				
Popsicles				

sources; peanut butter, dried beans, lentils, nuts, and soybean curd (tofu) are also high-protein foods. However, the latter foods, containing plant proteins, have certain nutritional limitations. Although their protein content per serving may be as high as that of animal protein (2 tablespoons of peanut butter contains as much protein as 7 ounces of milk or 1 ounce of tunafish), plant protein contains proportionally smaller amounts of certain essential amino acids than does animal protein (see Chapters 2 and 5 for a fuller discussion). This is not a nutritional problem if other protein foods containing high proportions of the missing essential amino acids are eaten at the same time. For example, if peanut butter is eaten on bread or with a glass of milk, all the essential amino acids are provided. However, peanut butter licked off the finger or spoon, with no other protein source, does not supply the needed essential amino acids.

> Tofu (bean curd) is a high-protein food that is rapidly becoming popular among vegetarians and people on macrobiotic diets. It has a soft, custard-like consistency and is relatively low in calories and very high in calcium. Although one essential amino acid, methionine, is found in lower amounts in tofu than in animal protein, tofu is usually eaten with grains or milk, and the missing essential amino acid is supplied by these foods. Since it takes on the flavor of anything with which it is combined, it is used for main dishes, salads, and desserts. The main advantages for the young eater are that it is sufficiently bland to satisfy the needs of young taste buds, can be eaten with a spoon, does not need to be chewed for long, and is easy to digest. (See ref. 4 for more information and recipes.)

Foods containing protein should be varied as frequently as possible so the many nutrients which "piggy-back" (i.e., are found along with the protein) are also supplied. For example, meat is a good source of thiamin, iron, zinc, vitamins B_{12} and B_6, and pantothenic acid. Eggs contain substantial amounts of phosphorus, sulfur, vitamin A, and iron (although the absorption of iron from eggs is not as good as its absorption from meat). However, children often place limits on the protein foods they eat. Meat tends to be unpopular because it may be too chewy or stringy. Lamb chops, however, seem to be highly acceptable to some 2-year-olds, who are unaware of their price. Fish often does not taste good to a young child, and if chicken is at all dry it may be hard for a toddler to swallow. (He often prefers to chew on it and then throw it on the floor. Dairy products and eggs are good alternative sources of protein; their texture and taste are usually acceptable, and they can be used as ingredients and/or main dishes in every meal.

Vitamins and Minerals

Children and adolescents require the same vitamins and minerals as adults: the amount needed increases with age and reaches its highest value during adolescence. Since it is necessary to eat a wide variety of foods to have an adequate intake of most vitamins and minerals, the limited food preferences of the child may result in inadequate consumption of these important nutrients. The teenager is just as vulnerable; the foods eaten during these years have moved beyond apple juice and toast but are just as limited in nutrient content (french fries, doughnuts, candy bars, potato chips, soft drinks) (Tables 4 and 5).

In order to improve the nutritional quality of their childrens' diet, many parents resort to buying snack foods fortified with some vitamins and minerals. Somehow buying a vitamin-enriched cupcake seems an easier way of getting nutrients into a child than coating a carrot with chocolate syrup. Table 6 lists the nutrient content of some of the better-known juvenile snack foods and drinks. The nutrient content of cereal with milk and a box of raisins is listed for comparison.

Although snack foods fortified with nutrients are probably better than a comparable unfortified product, they certainly are not a substitute for basic foods. Parents should be extra sensitive to advertisements that promote snack foods fortified with a couple of vitamins. They may be fine in an emergency but a steady diet of them leaves much to be desired nutritionally.

TABLE 4. *Day's food intake for two boys, age 12 and 14,*
in the same neighborhood (mid-August)

Time	12-Year-old	14-Year-old
9:30 a.m.	2 Plain doughnuts ½ Canteloupe	Orange juice (4 oz) 2 Bowls Cheerios (4 oz) 1 Glass milk (8 oz) 1 Banana 1 Vitamin pill (Unicap)
10:30	One vanilla soft ice cream cone	One vanilla soft ice cream cone
1:15 p.m.		Tunafish (3 oz) 1 Slice white bread Ovaltine (8 oz) Lemon meringue pie (1 slice) Chocolate chip ice cream (2 Tbs)
3:00	Hot dog 1 Can root beer	1 Can pepsi cola 1 Large soft ice cream cone
5:15	1 Chocolate chip cookie	Half popsicle
6:30		Spaghetti and meatballs (1 cup) Milk (16 oz) Ice cream (1 cup)
7:00	Bluefish (4 oz) French fries (1 cup) Carrots (6) Lettuce and tomato salad (small bowl) Milk (8 oz)	

TABLE 5. *Food intake of the two boys in Table 4 during the school year*

Meal	Food
12-Year-old	
Breakfast	Cereal (bran), milk, orange juice, toast
Lunch	School lunch: meat, potato, desert, chocolate milk
After school snack	Raw carrots and pretzels
Dinner	Meat, potato, salad, ice cream, milk
Evening	Two or three toaster pizza rounds and soda
14-Year-old	
Breakfast	Cereal (frosted flakes), milk, orange juice
Lunch	Prepared at home: one sandwich (usually tunafish or bologna), fruit, brownies or cookies, chocolate milk
After school snack	Popcorn, soda
Dinner	Meat, potato, salad, milk, ice cream

Neither admits to eating any cooked vegetables except when they eat Chinese food.

Vitamin A

Generations of children have been told that eating carrots will enable them to see in the dark, and bushels of this vegetable may have been consumed as a result. Unfortunately, eating large amounts of vitamin A-containing foods such as carrots does not guarantee the vision of an owl; however, the ability to see in dim and even normal light does depend on adequate amounts of this vitamin.

Vitamin A, in the form of the compound retinal, combines with a special protein in the cones and rods of the retina. (Cones are responsible for color vision and rods for black and white vision in dim light.) When light hits this retinal-protein structure its form changes slightly, and this results in a signal which is sent by the nerves to the visual center of the brain. As the retinal bound to the protein changes back to its original form (which occurs so the process can take place again), some of the retinal is used up. Its replacement requires vitamin A. If an unsufficient amount of this vitamin is stored in the body or is present in the diet, the used retinal is not completely replaced and the ability to see in dim light is gradually lost. One of the first signs of vitamin A deficiency is "nightblindness," i.e., difficulty seeing in dim light or prolonged adjustment to seeing in dim light after being in bright light.

Vitamin A is also necessary for the formation and maintenance of membranes that surround the body's cells and the membranes of structures inside cells. Without sufficient vitamin A, tissues such as the skin and the membranes which line the mouth, gastrointestinal, and urinary tracts, as well as the tissues of various glands, cannot remain intact.

Recently some evidence from work on cells grown in the laboratory has shown that the tissue which forms the skin (epithelial tissue) can develop potentially cancerous lesions when deprived of vitamin A. When vitamin A is supplied to these cells they recover and the abnormal precancerous cells are replaced by normal cells. It is hoped that further research will indicate whether use of vitamin A, in the form in which it is active in the body (retinoids), will prevent cancer from developing in parts of the body where precancerous lesions exist. However, the answer to this question is still many

TABLE 6. *Nutrient content of some snack foods[a]*

Food	Serving Size	Calories	Percent of recommended daily allowance (for adults)[b]								
			Protein	Vit. A	Vit. C	Riboflavin	Thiamin	Calcium	Iron	Niacin
Cherry Squoze (flavored fruit drink in powdered form)	8 fl oz	40	0	0	15	0	0	0	0	0
Crunchola (cereal-chocolate candy bar)	1 bar	160	10	0	0	6	6	2	6	0
Nature Valley Granola Bar (cereal-filled candy bar)	1 bar	110	4	0	0	2	6	2	4	0
Potato chips	15 chips	150	2	0	15	2	2	0	0	6
Cracker Jacks	1 box	120	2	0	6	6	0	2	4	4
Drink-a-doo (fruit drink concentrate)	6 oz	80	0	0	45	0	0	0	0	0
Chocolate food sticks (taffy-like candy stick)[c]	4 sticks	180	6	6	6	6	6	6	6	6
Devil dogs	1 package (4 bites)	200	4	0	0	8	10	2	10	0
Sugar smacks plus whole milk[d]	1 oz} 4 oz}	190	10	30	2	35	25	15	2	25
Raisins[e]	½ box (302)	250	4	4	0	2	0	4	6	2

[a]This nutrient information is available from package labels.
[b]One hundred percent of the Recommended Daily Allowance (RDA) of a particular nutrient satisfies the daily adult requirement for that nutrient.
[c]Also contain 6% of RDA for vitamins E, D, B_6, B_{12}; folic acid; phosphorus; iodine; and magnesium.
[d]Also contains 25% of the RDA for B_6, B_{12}, folic acid, and vitamin D.
[e]Also contains 10% of the RDA for copper.

years away and does *not* justify eating excessive amounts of vitamin A, especially since large quantities are *known* to be harmful.

Vitamin A does not have to be eaten every day because the body is able to store it. Vitamin A-containing foods should be eaten several times a week, however. Vitamin A is found in dairy products (e.g., milk, cheese, butter); it is present as another compound, beta-carotene, in many fruits and vegetables. Watermelon, nectarines, peaches, tomatoes, cantaloupe, broccoli, carrots, romaine and other lettuce, spinach, sweet potatoes (and yams), winter and acorn squash all contain substantial amounts of this vitamin.[1]

However, despite its widespread availability in food, it is still possible to eat a vitamin A-deficient diet; surveys have shown that children and adolescents in certain parts of the country do not get enough of this vitamin (3). A high-carbohydrate diet that includes very few dairy products or vegetables can easily lead to a deficient vitamin A intake.

Vitamin A can be added to the diet easily and inexpensively. Powdered dry milk solids are usually fortified with this vitamin, do not cost much, and can be added to a variety of foods (cake batters, pancake mix, meatloaf, mashed potatoes). Cheese, margarine, or butter are often used as ingredients, and bread and butter or bread and cheese are often eaten by children who would not touch a carrot. Certain vegetables and fruits high in vitamin A are relatively inexpensive and can be included as ingredients in several dishes. Carrots can be concealed in stews, meatloaf, tunafish salad, and even baked into breads and cakes, although children tend to get suspicious when a piece of cake has orange flecks in it. Raw carrots are good with peanut butter on them. During the summer, at least, many types of fruits (e.g., watermelon, cantaloupe, peaches, nectarines, apricots) can supply vitamin A. The winter season limits the number of vitamin A-containing fruits to those such as prunes (which are becoming more respectable) and bananas (although they have only a moderate amount of this vitamin). Apples, unfortunately, do not contain much vitamin A (one peach contains nine times the vitamin A of one apple).

A few years ago vitamin A was promoted as a cure for skin problems, and some teenagers who tend to be afflicted with more than their share of skin worries started to eat massive doses. The problem is that excessive amounts of vitamin A can be harmful; some of the more unpleasant side effects include abdominal discomfort, fatigue, brittle nails, headaches, and, ironically, dry, scaly skin (5).

Vitamin D

Vitamin D participates in the process of calcium absorption from the intestinal tract into the bloodstream. Sunlight (see Chapter 6) and vitamin D-fortified foods

---

[1]Excellent sources of vitamin A include kale, collard greens, apricots, persimmons, pigweed, dandelion greens, and Swiss chard. However, many people do not eat these foods, or do so infrequently, because they are unfamiliar tasting and looking, are hard to find in supermarkets, or their methods of preparation are unknown.

(e.g., milk) provide enough vitamin D to eliminate the problem of deficiency among most children and teenagers. However, rickets, caused by lack of vitamin D and thought to be practically nonexistent today, has been found with some frequency among children of strict vegetarians and members of the macrobiotic community. These children are not fed dairy products; and since the climate often restricts the number of days in which the skin can be exposed to the sun, they have no way of obtaining sufficient vitamin D without using some form of supplementation. One pediatrician in the Boston area routinely prescribes codliver oil (very high in vitamin D) for all the macrobiotic children he sees.

Vitamin K

Coagulation of the blood depends on vitamin K; unless this vitamin is present, several proteins that participate in forming a blood clot are not produced. (For the child who spends half his leisure time having cuts and scrapes bandaged, this vitamin can be very useful.) About 50% of the vitamin K we need is produced by certain harmless bacteria that live in our intestines; the rest comes from foods such as green vegetables (lettuce, broccoli), meats, butter, cheese, and even coffee and green tea.

Vitamin E

The need for vitamin E depends primarily on the amount of polyunsaturated fats[2] in the diet. Over the past two decades the American diet has changed from one high in saturated fats (butter, lard, chicken fat, shortening) to one using a substantial amount of unsaturated fats (vegetable oils and margarines made from vegetable oil). This increase in polyunsaturated fats has caused an increase in our need for vitamin E; fortunately, the vegetable oils and dairy products are a good source of vitamin E, along with poultry, meat, fish, and wheat germ (not apt to be a daily favorite among the younger set). Hence it is difficult to avoid eating foods that contain vitamin E even if the selection of foods is limited.

Vitamin E, also known as tocopherol, has been endowed with great powers by many food faddists. Supposedly, vitamin E cures ailments ranging from infertility to old age (6). Although there is no evidence available to confirm these claims, tocopherols (there are several types) do have an important function in the body's biochemistry.

> Polyunsaturated fatty acids are found in compounds called phospholipids. Phospholipids are important structural components of the membrane that surrounds cells and the membranes that surround small structures within the cell. The unsaturated parts of a polyunsaturated fatty acid can be changed by oxygen (always present in the cell) into a substance called a free radical. These free radicals

---

[2]Polyunsaturate: On each fatty acid molecule there are many places to which a hydrogen atom can be attached. Saturated fats have hydrogen atom at each of these places; poly (meaning many) *un*saturated fats lack hydrogen atoms at many of these locations.

apparently can damage the structural parts of the cell. Vitamin E prevents the oxidation of the unsaturated fatty acids and so protects the cell from damage from these free radicals.

some recent reports claim that vitamin E may protect the lungs against damage from air pollutants such as ozone (found in smog) by preventing the ozone from oxidizing the polyunsaturated compounds in our lung cells (7). This has not been conclusively proved, however.

The exact amount of vitamin E needed by adults and children is not known since it varies with the amount of polyunsaturated fats in the diet. The levels set forth in the Recommended Dietary Allowance (1979) (Table 1) are considered adequate, and vitamin E deficiency has been found only among children who suffer from a rare inability to absorb dietary fat.

Some teenagers consume large quantities of vitamin E, rub it on their faces, or wash their hair with it in the belief that their hair will be glossy and their skin smooth. (Adults sometimes consume the vitamin in excess amounts or rub it on to prevent wrinkles.) Washing one's hair or face in soybean oil, which is very high in vitamin E, produces oily hair or skin, nothing else. There is no evidence, despite claims to the contrary, that vitamin E will remove wrinkles from anything, even a prune.

Thiamin (B₁)

Thiamin participates in a series of cellular reactions that transfer energy contained in food such as bread to specific compounds which hold energy in a form the cell can use. Thiamin is also needed for the synthesis of the nucleic acids DNA and RNA, which are essential to life.

Calorie consumption determines, to some extent, the amount of thiamin needed by the body. As caloric consumption increases, so does the need for thiamin. In fact, the requirement for this vitamin is usually expressed as so much per 1,000 calories. An adolescent who consumes food like a vacuum cleaner needs more thiamin than a 2 year old who buries his food in a flower pot. For example a 15-year-old boy needs three times as much thiamin (1.5 mg) as a 2-year-old (0.5 mg).

Some of the food sources of thiamin are listed in the nursery rhyme "Oats, peas, beans, and barley grow." However, if oatmeal, barley, or split peas are not everyday fare, alternatives are available. Dry cereals that are fortified (check labels), enriched flour products (e.g., pancake mix, bread, muffins), enriched pasta (macaroni, spaghetti), and meat are good sources of thiamin. Some nuts and seeds contain substantial amounts: peanuts, pecans, sunflower seeds. The common pea is an excellent source of thiamin, a fortunate occurrence since peas are usually one of the few vegetables children enjoy. Soybeans are also a good source of thiamin and recently have become somewhat popular among teenagers. Beans such as those used for baked beans and chili (kidney, pea, or navy beans) also contain thiamin.

Riboflavin (B_2)

Like thiamin, riboflavin participates in enzymatic reactions in the cells (it is called a coenzyme) and is involved in many of the same energy-producing reactions. Meat and dairy products contain ample amounts of riboflavin; the teenager who drinks a quart of milk with his afternoon snack more than satisfies his B_2 requirements (two glasses of milk contain the B_2 needs of a young child). Other dairy products (e.g., cottage cheese, yogurt, hard cheese) are also excellent sources of this vitamin. Other relatively good sources of B_2 include mushrooms, cocoa, watermelon, eggs, eels, oysters, and frog legs. Fortunately eggs, cocoa, and watermelon are common items in the diets of children; the other foods, with the exception of mushrooms, are apt to be eaten infrequently if at all by Americans under or over 18.

Riboflavin deficiency has been found among poor children and adolescents, perhaps because of the expense of meat and the avoidance of milk by some ethnic groups. Lactose intolerance, discussed in Chapter 6, develops during childhood; many studies of the milk-drinking habits of elementary school-age children with this condition reveal a drastic drop in milk consumption. (A lactose-free milk is now available in some parts of the country. It is called acidophilus-treated milk and contains lactose already broken down into the simple sugars: glucose and galactose, thus rendering it suitable for those with lactose intolerance.)

Children often avoid milk simply because they prefer to drink something else. Soft drinks are being consumed in increasingly greater quantities, and this trend is accelerated by the presence of soft drink machines in many schools. Indeed some school systems are removing their vending machines in order to increase milk consumption in the school cafeteria. In addition, a recent report indicated that milk consumption among elementary school children (8) increased significantly when the children are allowed to choose chocolate-flavored milk; when they could drink only unflavored milk, they drank much less. Perhaps making chocolate milk available is the only effective way of "weaning" kids from soft drinks. This may not work, however, with calorie-conscious teenagers who do not want to "waste their calories" on milk of any type and so drink diet soft drinks instead. (Do they realize that water has no calories?)

The young child who goes through periods of avoiding meat and milk (and cottage cheese, yogurt, and hard cheese) may not obtain a sufficient amount of riboflavin in his diet. (Eating less than two-thirds of the RDA for a nutrient is considered an insufficient intake.) However, a mother can surreptitiously add milk in a powdered or evaporated form to many foods (by wrapping the box or can in brown paper the child does not realize she is adding milk). Evaporated milk added to pancake batter, cake mixes, and puddings provides riboflavin in a concentrated form so that even small portions contain substantial amounts.

Lastly, skipping meals and snacking, activities not limited to any age group, can easily lead to a deficiency of riboflavin. Snack foods rarely include pot roast, mushrooms, or cottage cheese. The recent trend to yogurt eating, however, may aid in providing riboflavin to chronic snackers.

> Last spring I saw three 10-year-old boys stop at a small grocery store to buy fruit-flavored yogurt for a snack after a ball game—a good sign that the yogurt trend may be catching on among the unwashed-neck set.

Niacin (B₃)

Niacin also acts as a coenzyme in the cells. It forms part of a compound that is essential to certain biochemical reactions, e.g., those involved in forming energy-containing substances or in synthesizing fatty acids. Dietary niacin deficiency is rare among children and adolescents since the vitamin is found in many foods. Moreover, niacin can be made by the body from the essential amino acid tryptophan. Most flour and cereal products are enriched with niacin, providing a reliable, constant source of this vitamin. After all, few people consistently avoid cakes, waffles, breakfast cereals, muffins, bread, and pastas. Although dairy products contain only small amounts of niacin, the protein in these foods and other animal protein foods (eggs, meat, and fish) is a good source of tryptophan and ultimately niacin. Among commonly eaten vegetables, peas, potatoes (even potato chips), corn on the cob, and beans (white and red) are also good sources. Peanuts and peanut butter contain substantial amounts of B_3.

Pyridoxal Phosphate (B₆)

Vitamin B_6 is needed for a large variety of biochemical reactions. It is the coenzyme for more than 60 enzymatic reactions, including the synthesis of certain amino acids that do not have to be supplied in the diet, formation of neurotransmitters (compounds that transmit messages between brain cells), production of niacin from tryptophan, and conversion of the stored form of glucose (glycogen) into glucose itself.

The vitamin requirement increases with age and is also partially related to the amount of protein in the diet. Some older adolescents who routinely consume enormous amounts of protein may need 0.5 to 1 mg more vitamin B_6 than the average eater.

> An 18-year-old college freshman who kept a record of his weekly food consumption ate what he termed a "normal amount of food for his peer group." He ate the following amounts of protein foods in 2 days: 8 ounces of tunafish, 2 ounces of American cheese, 48 ounces of milk, 3 hot dogs, 1 lb of roast lamb, 1 lb of steak. His average daily protein intake was 166 grams; the RDA for his age group is 60 grams per day. Clearly his vitamin B_6 needs must be increased by this large (one might say excessive) protein consumption.

B_6 is supplied in a variety of foods likely to be eaten by children and adolescents. Peanuts and peanut butter, bananas, corn flakes, potatoes, raisins, rice (or rice pudding with raisins), peas, chicken, and wheat germ are all good sources of this vitamin. (Wheat germ can be mixed into many foods, from pancakes to hamburger, without much chance of detection.) However, dieting often eliminates many of these B_6-containing foods; it is therefore advisable to check any sort of restricted food intake for vitamin B_6 sufficiency.

Folic Acid

Beef liver, brewers' yeast, and cow peas are all excellent sources of folic acid, as are beet and mustard greens, soy flour, cooked wheat cereals, and kale. However, the typical American child or teenager is unlikely to eat these foods frequently or at all. Asparagus—fresh, frozen, or canned—is a good source of folic acid, but it is an expensive vegetable and the taste may not be acceptable to a young child. Folic acid is also found in a wide variety of other foods but in such small amounts that large quantities of these foods must be eaten to meet the folic acid requirements. (The function of folic acid is discussed in Chapter 5.)

Some of the folic acid-containing foods eaten by children include peanuts, peanut butter, lettuce, peas, spinach, broccoli, and whole wheat bread (wheat germ is also a good source). When the characteristically limited diet of children and teenagers results in low folic acid intake, one solution is to offer the child or teenager a breakfast cereal fortified with the vitamin. (Many of the multivitamin-fortified cereals contain folic acid.) Breakfast cereals need not be eaten only in the morning, and they make snacks that are nutritionally superior to cookies or candy.

Vitamin B_{12}

Vitamin B_{12}, unlike folic acid, is relatively easy to include in the diet since it is found in meat, fish, dairy products, and eggs. Indeed only the diets of strict vegetarians who eat no dairy products or eggs lack this vitamin. However, families who follow this way of eating can eat cereals fortified with vitamin B_{12} or drink B_{12}-fortified soy milk.

Ascorbic Acid (Vitamin C)

Although the association between vitamin C (ascorbic acid) and the prevention or cure for the common cold no longer appears very firm, vitamin C does have some well-established, important functions. Ascorbic acid is involved in the formation of collagen, a structural component of bones, teeth, and connective tissue (the tissue that supports muscles and organs and which forms first in the healing of cuts or wounds). When vitamin C is absent, wounds do not heal well and small hemorrhages appear in parts of the body. Scurvy, the vitamin C deficiency disease, was extremely common among children and adults until this century, even though it was recognized that certain foods would prevent this disease. Poverty, popular ignorance, and unavailability of these foods prevented many people from consuming enough vitamin C. In his book *The Good Old Days—They were Terrible* (9), Otto Bettman describes a diet common to settlers of the American West as consisting of "corn, corn, and salted hogmeat." Scurvy was a natural result of this diet.

Fortunately, modern methods of preserving and transporting foods have made vitamin C-rich foods abundantly available to everyone. Citrus fruits in the winter; watermelon, tomatoes, and strawberries in the summer; and potatoes, green peppers, and cabbages all year round are good sources of this vitamin. For those who like to drink their vitamins, natural and fabricated fruit juices containing vitamin C (added by nature or the manufacturer) are another common source of this vitamin in the American diet. It is important to note, though, that natural fruit juices contain nutrients besides vitamin C: potassium, phosphorus, thiamin, riboflavin, niacin, magnesium, and vitamin A. Juices made from water, artificial flavor, color, and ascorbic acid cost less than natural juices, but they contain no other nutrients, unless the water is fluoridated.

Minerals

Mothers who have preschool children with eating problems or older children who consume haphazard diets often give them vitamin supplements to fill in some of the nutritional gaps. Although multivitamin pills do compensate for a *vitamin*-deficient diet, they hardly ever provide any essential *minerals* other than iron (check the labels). Therefore the mother who says she does not worry about what her children eat because she gives them a vitamin pill every day" is deluding herself. If children are obviously not eating a nutritionally complete diet, and supplementation with a vitamin preparation seems appropriate, then a supplement that contains a variety of minerals (e.g., zinc, calcium, magnesium, iron) should be chosen. Another solution may be to "convince" your children to eat a cereal supplemented with multivitamins and minerals. These cereals contain several minerals; they are not a substitute for a varied and nutritionally adequate diet but are useful (if eaten) during periods of insufficient nutrient consumption such as trips, eating rebellions, dieting, skipping meals, and excessive snacking.

> One way to promote a nutritious cereal is by conveniently forgetting to buy any other kind. After a few days of vehement protest, the cereal will be tried. For the young child who likes cereal for its prizes rather than taste, buying a few trinkets and putting them at the bottom of the box may stimulate interest in his eating his way down to them.

Growth requires an adequate supply of dietary minerals, especially those such as *calcium* and *phosphorus,* which help form the skeleton. The eating habits of children and adolescents, however, sometimes eliminate certain minerals from the diet or decrease their absorption into the circulation from the intestine. For example, the amount of calcium eaten should be equal to the amount of phosphorus in order for calcium to be absorbed efficiently. However, eating habits typical of today's child are preventing this from happening. One such habit is the rapid decline in milk consumption and its replacement by enormous consumption of soft drinks. The causes for this are evident. Advertising has convinced a large segment of the entire population (not merely children and teenagers) that "everything goes better with..." or that "a hamburger and french fries call for a..." or that "in order to be a youthful swinger who does not fall off a water ski, you should drink a...." Reinforcing this trend is the proliferation of soft drink vending machines in schools (usually resulting in an immediate decline in milk consumption at the cafeteria), the availability of low-calorie soft drinks, and the unavailability of milk at some fast-food restaurants. Hence unless calcium is obtained from other dietary products (e.g., cheese, yogurt, cottage cheese, or ice cream), children and teenagers do not get enough of it. Furthermore, because soft drinks contain large quantities of phosphorus, the ratio of calcium to phosphorus in the diet may go way down if soft drinks are consumed in large quantity, making it more difficult for the little calcium that is consumed to be absorbed.

The effects of this problem may last well beyond adolescence. The American way of eating has produced a soft drink-consuming public; and if the habit of drinking milk is lost around the time the baby comes off the bottle, the baby may grow up to be someone who continues to obtain insufficient calcium throughout life. Chronically insufficient calcium is one of the nutritional factors that seems to be related to diseases such as osteoporosis in the elderly (10).

One solution to this may be to switch solutions. In cases of dire thirst, most people will drink any handy liquid. The refrigerator is usually the first place a child looks for a drink (water is considered good only for bathing and washing the dog); if milk is the only liquid residing in the refrigerator, then it is usually drunk. Children living under these "austere" conditions may even discover the joy of a cold glass of milk with a cookie. It takes time, but eventually the soda-drinking habit loses its grip on young taste buds, and a day may come when the child or teenager prefers milk or even water!

Zinc participates in many essential enzymatic reactions, including one which enables carbon dioxide to be carried by the blood to the lungs, where it is eliminated. (Carbon dioxide is produced by the cells during the conversion of nutrients to chemical energy.) Zinc also maintains the structure of the nucleic acids (RNA and DNA) which direct and participate in protein synthesis.

Children of low-income families, or those with severely limited tastes, may find it difficult to obtain sufficient amounts of zinc. A recent study of a group of 3-to 4-year-old low-income children enrolled in a Head Start program revealed that these children were shorter than 90% of their age group and had low body stores of zinc (11). Their decreased growth rate was considered to be due to the low zinc levels in their diet.

Although zinc is found in many foods, the best sources of it are expensive, not eaten by children, or both. Shellfish (e.g., lobster, oysters, crabs) are good sources of zinc, as are nuts, red meat, and pork. Cheese is a fair source, along with chili con carne, tunafish, garlic, chocolate, oatmeal, and soups (canned or homemade) containing some meat. Wheat germ is an excellent source of this mineral. Fruits and vegetables have a low zinc content.

Finicky eaters, vegetarians, and dieting teenagers may not eat much zinc; however, adding wheat germ covertly to the food of the first, including nuts in the diet of the second, and serving shellfish (very low in calories) to the third may help supply some of this necessary nutrient.

Iron deficiency has been and continues to be a major nutritional problem among children in the United States according to a recent survey (3). In fact, iron tends to be deficient in the diets of many Americans regardless of age; the limited amount and variety of food eaten by children simply exacerbates a common problem.

Unfortunately, many foods that contain iron (spinach, eggs, oatmeal) also contain compounds that bind to iron and prevent it from being absorbed efficiently (see Chapter 5 for further discussion). Meats supply iron in the most concentrated and easily absorbed form. Organ meats (liver, sweetbreads, kidneys) contain the most iron, but, to put it politely, these foods are not favored by children. Usually the first confrontation between mother and child is over liver, and often the only winner is the local cat or dog. (Alligator meat is also very high in iron.) Beef, veal, lamb, and pork are the second best sources of this mineral; poultry contains considerably less.

Although certain vegetables (beans, chickpeas, lentils, soybeans) contain absorbable iron, it is not absorbed *as well* from these foods as from meat. Apparently the iron-containing substance called heme, which is found in meat, gets into the bloodstream more efficiently than does the iron from plant foods. Some studies have shown that eating meat along with other iron-containing foods (e.g., beans) promotes the absorption of iron from the nonmeat sources. Ascorbic acid also enhances iron absorption, so theoretically putting ketchup (which contains some vitamin C) on a hamburger may be nutritionally beneficial. Sunflower seeds and pumpkin seeds contain as much iron as meat, and like roasted soybeans, can be used as snack foods. (There is no written law that says snacks have to be nonnutritious.) Raisins, prunes, dates, and dried apricots are also good sources of iron; and since they are sweet and chewy, do not melt in the hand or mouth, and fit into pockets nicely, they are handy ways of getting this somewhat evasive nutrient into the diet. It is unfortunate that these products are not more accessible as snack items in fast-food restaurants, vending machines, or school cafeterias, or (with the exception of raisins) are not packaged in small lunch bag quantities the way potato chips or cheese curls are.

Iron deficiency is most common among teenage girls, their peculiar eating habits and regular loss of blood through menstruation contributing to the situation. However, getting a teenage girl to stop dieting or start eating prunes instead of french fries is almost as difficult as getting a 2-year-old to eat liver. Two good sources of iron, meat and iron-fortified cereals, are often avoided because they are "too high in calories" or "too dull." In addition, vegetarians and young vegetarian sympathizers often avoid red meat because of its undeniable animal-like properties.

Changing the eating habits of teenagers through traditional educational means is rarely successful. Advertisements in magazines or television programs directed toward this age group may be the only effective means of altering their food habits. The profits gained from the teenage market attest to the success of advertising; hence it may be possible to utilize this medium to promote the acceptance of, for instance, iron-fortified foods or supplements. After all, if advertisements can convince a teenage girl to use pimple remedies or hair conditioners, they may be able to convince her to eat certain foods.

The other minerals required by the child and teenager are widely distributed in foods and are easy to obtain. *Iodine* is a partial exception to this. It does not occur naturally in foods grown away from coastal areas, and until recently the only reliable source was iodized (iodine-supplemented) salt. Iodine is now being added to many processed foods as well. If plain salt is used instead of iodized salt, it is necessary to read the labels of all other food products to see if iodized salt is an ingredient. Alternatively, sea salt, which is found in health food stores (and costs considerably more than iodized salt), can be used. The safest and most reliable way of getting this essential mineral into the bodies of your children is to depend on salt fortified with iodine.

EATING PATTERNS DURING CHILDHOOD AND ADOLESCENCE

During childhood and adolescence an individual syle of eating takes shape, influenced first by the family, local customs, and religious and ethnic traditions, and subsequently by peers, advertisements, and experiences in school, camp, and restaurants. Everyone accepts or rejects many foods as an adult because of childhood associations, and the influence of these memories is often so subtle it goes unrecognized unless attention is drawn to a particular food habit.

Recently in a college seminar students analyzed some of their feelings about particular foods.

> An Orthodox Jewish student could not bring himself to taste an imitation bacon product made from soybeans. He knew the imitation bacon was kosher, but it smelled so much like the bacon he had learned was a forbidden food when he was very young that the thought of eating it made him feel sick.
> Another student told how her family had deliberately cultivated a preference for the dark meat of turkey in her younger brother. The rest of the family preferred white meat, so they conspired to make him believe, when he was very young, that dark meat

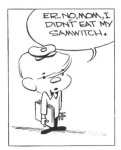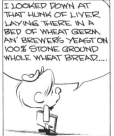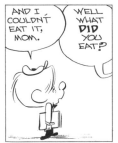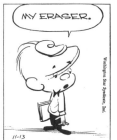

(© Washington Star Syndicate, Inc.)

was better and special, and that they were allowing him to eat it because he was so special. He grew up believing that white meat is inferior to dark and has never eaten it.

During early childhood a large number of foods are introduced into the diet and usually accepted. Slightly later, during the preschool and elementary school years, a neophobia develops (12) toward unfamiliar foods. This is characterized by a preference for familiar foods, reluctance to try new foods, and difficulty, even as an adult, in accepting foods alien to one's culture. Even adults tend to feel comfortable with certain components of a meal and expect these foods to be present at most meals. A dinner of meat, a starch food (bread, potatoes, pasta, or rice), and a salad and/or familiar cooked vegetables is typical of many meals in the United States. (An acquaintance of mine told me that her family ate meat and mashed potatoes for supper every single day while she was growing up; she never had such exotic items as carrots or string beans until she went to college.) Many Americans would feel uncomfortable if they were confronted with a bowl of rice, a plate of raw fish, pickled seaweed, and a cucumber with vinegar salad for dinner.

Regardless of the sophistication of our palate, we ultimately return to the foods with which we are most familiar. Travelers abroad who accept new and usually extremely palatable food eventually long for some "simple American food." It is as if we learn a language of food around the time we are learning to speak. Just as we feel most comfortable speaking our own language, so too we feel the most content when eating foods familiar since childhood.

Many food preferences and aversions learned during childhood are passed on to the next generation. For example, a parent may not state publically that he dislikes liver, but if he obviously does not eat it when it is served, his aversion will be noted by his children and perhaps incorporated into their own patterns of food likes and dislikes. Children may also develop aversions to foods because of unfamiliarity. If certain foods were not served at home when they are young, they may never bring themselves to try these foods when they are adults.

> A youngster came into my kitchen one day as I was skinning an eggplant. "What's that?" he asked. When I told him it was an eggplant, he looked very dubious and said, "I wouldn't eat something that looks like that."

Parents tend to rank foods in order of importance. Certain foods take on a reward value and are offered as inducements to eat other foods or as rewards for good behavior. There is usually no relationship between the nutrient content of food and desirability; that is, potato chips, soda, cupcakes, and ice cream sundaes are usually considered more desirable than cottage cheese, carrots, and toast. (Notice how often the phrase "treat yourself" appears in advertisements as an inducement for adults to buy sweets or snack foods.) Other foods may be ranked as worthy of important occasions. Steaks, turkeys, lobsters, and roast beef tend to be foods reserved for special occasions. Food with similar protein content such as tunafish, hamburger, and stew meat are not considered as worthy and are usually served more frequently. Obviously expense is an important factor in determining how important a food is, and should the cost of tunafish rise as rapidly as that of coffee, for example, it may become as special a food as caviar.

An adult usually moves away from his parents' perceptions of important and unimportant foods only when he adds to his eating repertoire foods which were never eaten in his parents' home. How, for example, does one rank bean curd, oysters, or buckwheat groats according to childhood perceptions of the status of foods if these were never eaten during childhood?

A special word about vegetables: Many adults rarely eat vegetables because they disliked them as children. Often the basis for the dislike was their method of preparation.

> A woman from the South said that she had always thought vegetables must be cooked for 2 hours until they attained a mush-like consistency. As an adult, she moved to another part of the country and discovered the "stir-fry" method of cooking vegetables, which leaves them slightly undercooked and crisp. They tasted like a new food to her.
>
> A group of teenage boys affirmed their dislike for home-cooked vegetables also; they said they ate only potatoes, corn on the cob, and salads at home. However, when asked what they do with the vegetables that accompany many dishes in a Chinese restaurant, they said they always eat those vegetables because "they don't taste like vegetables—they taste good."

Maybe it is time to change our traditional ways of cooking vegetables.

The emotional associations the child makes with food and eating continue to affect his food choices and, to some extent, his control over food intake during adulthood. This topic is discussed further in the chapter on obesity (Chapter 4). The point is that eating habits do not merely emerge. They are learned and therefore can be at least partially taught.

Ideally, children and adolescents form eating styles that include an almost automatic choice of nutritionally correct foods and an awareness that these foods should be eaten routinely. This is not a totally unattainable objective. If children routinely eat dairy products, citrus fruits or juices, vegetables and fruits, cereals, salads, meat, chicken, eggs, and cheese, these foods become expected parts of meals and are missed if they are not available for any length of time. For such children, a lengthy diet of junk food quickly loses its appeal. A friend decided to stop cooking for a week while her husband was away on business and toured the various fast food franchises on a local highway. After a few days of fried chicken, milk shakes, hamburgers, and french fries, her children demanded that she make them a real dinner with vegetables, salad, fruits, and milk. Meanwhile, her husband, frustrated by the lack of fresh vegetables on airplanes and at conferences, had taken to scavenging the garnishes from buffet tables whenever he went to a reception: 5 minutes after his arrival, the platters would be denuded of all decoration.

Many records of food consumption over a week-long period have shown that people who have a consistently adequate nutrient intake manage to select foods over a week that satisfy their nutrient needs. They may not eat perfectly every day, but they usually compensate on one day for the deficiencies of another. How does this nutritional sense develop? It seems possible that children begin to acquire this sensitivity to their nutrient needs if they have access to a variety of nutritious foods while growing up. A toddler does not innately know that a carrot is considered less desirable than a candy bar by older children; and if carrots, dried fruits, or whole wheat bread are the only available snack foods, they will be eaten. A toddler is neither mature enough nor corrupted enough to say, "No thanks, I'll wait until we go out and then have some ice cream." Hence raising a child in a nutritionally sound eating environment increases the likelihood that nutritious foods, rather than junk foods, will come to mind when he is hungry.

> It also, however, may make it hard to keep babysitters. One teenager, returning from a household where the kitchen was stocked with yogurt, dried fruit, wheat germ, and fresh vegetables, claimed that she would never sit for that family again because there was nothing to eat.

Obviously, it is impossible to keep a child in a nutritionally pure environment for very long. Grandparents are likely to seduce the child's taste buds with ice cream, cookies, cake, candy, and potato chips; and many grandchildren fall under the influence of homemade chocolate chip cookies. Friends, nursery school birthday parties, teenage baby sitters who bring their own food, and various salespersons are also sources of good-tasting but nutritionally defective foods; and often it is politically unwise for the mother to refuse the food or lecture its donor on its lack of nutritional value. However, these occasional outside encounters with snack foods need not discourage a parent from restricting their consumption at home. Remember: out of sight, out of stomach. A child will continue to snack on nutritious foods at home if no others are available.

Television advertising is probably the most persistent force undermining good eating habits. After all, the current generation of grandmothers may be pursuing a career rather than baking cookies; and nursery school teachers are promoting yogurt these days; but television advertisements are still here, telling youngsters that if they eat yummy, crunchy, gooey things they can grow up and play with plastic toys that come inside cereal packages. Many consumer advocate organizations such as Action for Children's Television[3] are attempting to reduce or eliminate these advertisements. One sign of change in this direction is the increase in advertisements that promote well-balanced breakfasts and foods, e.g., bananas, grapes, and milk. However, these messages tend to be overwhelmed by the huge number of ads for junk foods that appear during prime TV time for children (e.g., Saturday morning).

There are several ways of combating the influence of television, and each should be tried; otherwise any attempt to inject some kind of nutritional sense into a child's eating habits will be doomed.

---

[3]Action for Children's Television, 46 Austin Street, Newtonville, Massachusetts 02160.

1. A young child can be told that his family simply does not eat the foods advertised on television. If this is stated positively and consistently to a young child and reinforced by never buying these foods and restricting his opportunities to eat them outside the home, the child is likely to accept these restrictions. Many children accept other types of food restrictions without question. Orthodox Jewish children accept the fact that they do not eat pork or shellfish, cannot mix dairy products with meat products, and avoid bread during Passover. Greek Orthodox children accept considerable dietary limitations during Lent. As mentioned earlier, these restrictions often become so ingrained in children that, as adults, they may actually get sick if they discover they have inadvertently eaten something which is forbidden.

2. Going to the supermarket without the child is another way of avoiding purchases of advertised nonnutritious food. Often the cost of a babysitter is less than the foods demanded by the child in the shopping cart or the cost of an uneaten supper due to late afternoon snacking.

3. If taking the child is unavoidable, then shop after, not before, a meal or snack. If putting nutritionally inferior items in the shopping cart is also unavoidable, piling them surreptitiously on the magazine rack next to the checkout counter when the child is not looking allows the parent to get home without actually buying these foods.

4. Restricting the child's TV viewing reduces the amount of exposure to the nonnutritious food advertisements. However, it does not eliminate them, and even short exposure to a novel food with "kid appeal" may be hard to resist. Under such circumstances, the mother can blunt the appeal of the advertisement by her own reactions. For example, she can pretend to gag at such foods as multicolored cereals and say "Who would *want* to eat green, yellow, orange, and red cereal with marshmallow centers?" (If the answer is "me," the battle has probably been lost.) If there is an animal in the house, the mother can ask the child if it would be good for the dog or cat to eat chocolate cupcakes with creamy centers rather than dog or cat food. Pet foods are advertised so frequently on television that most children understand the necessity of feeding a pet nutritious foods. If he perceives that Twinkies are not as good for the pet as pet food, then he can be asked why he thinks they are good for him.

5. Nothing is gained from buying nonnutritious foods and then fighting with the child over when they should be eaten. If the foods are in the house, the parents must expect that the child may want them instead of celery or apples and will want more of them than he should eat. Moreover, such foods should never be offered as rewards for eating nutritious foods or witheld as punishment. If these foods acquire value because they are considered treats or handed out grudgingly, the child can develop a craving or compulsive desire for them. It is better not to buy such foods at all or, if they are bought, to avoid making them special in any way.

6. Finally, ban Halloween! The last night in October can turn even the most nutritionally sensible child into a candy junkie. Since parents are warned to prevent their children from accepting food that is not commercially wrapped,

apples, homemade granola cookies, or figs cannot be given away. Boxed raisins are about the only nutritious treat one can hand out; and judging from the looks on the faces of children leaving our door, raisins are regarded as something closer to a trick than a treat.

In summary then, parents of children and adolescents must provide the nutrients needed to support rapid growth and development and create an eating environment in which nutritionally sensible eating habits are learned and adopted. No individual—child, adolescent, or adult—is going to make nutritionally perfect food choices every day, and fortunately our bodies are able to sustain several days of nutritionally inappropriate eating. (Car trips, bad colds, staying with a friend for a weekend or on the beach all day often result in a diet unadorned by vegetables, fruits, milk, or cereal.) However, unlike the adult, the child and adolescent must obtain nutrients for growth as well as for the maintenance of body functions, and he should not be allowed to follow an eating style that continually avoids foods with nutrient content.

The following techniques are offered as methods for improving the nutritional quality of the diet and food habits of the child and adolescent.

1. Keep track of what the child is eating. Do this as the child moves from one stage of development and life style to another. His eating habits change as he progresses from an at-home toddler to day-care centers or nursery school, when he enters elementary school, and again as his after-school activities become more elaborate and independent, and finally as he enters and proceeds through adolescence.

2. Anticipate periods when the child or teenager is apt to be hungry and be sure to have nutritious foods rather than nutritionally empty snack foods available. If the elementary school child is hungry when he comes home in the afternoon (probably because he threw away his lunch), serve him another lunch or even dinner if it is ready. (Preparing extra food the day before to be eaten as leftovers works well, especially if dinner is served late.) Make breakfast for the teenager at 10 PM when he takes a break from his homework; he probably will sleep through it in the morning. Bring along parts of lunch for the preschooler (fruit, cheese, half a sandwich) when you take him home from the playground, play group, or nursery school. He will be hungry then but may be too tired to eat when he arrives home. Feeding him his lunch in segments—some on the way home (in the car or on the tricycle) and some after his nap—prevents him from filling up on snack foods during these periods instead of the nutritious foods he needs.

3. Buy the foods you want your children to eat. Do not buy 4 gallons of soda and then complain because no one drinks milk.

4. Add nutritionally dense ingredients to whatever you cook if they cannot be detected, or alter the taste or quality of the food. (Wheat germ, evaporated or powdered milk, bananas, carrots, bran, oatmeal, raisins, eggs, cheese, and even sesame or sunflower seeds are examples of foods to add.) A list of edible sources of nutrients is found in Table 6.

5. Finally, set a good example. Do not let your own nutritional sins be passed on to your children. Eat breakfast with the family if you want them to eat this meal;

TABLE 6. *Edible sources of vitamins and minerals*

Vitamin A	Carrots, watermelon, nectarines, peaches, tomatoes, canteloupe, pumpkin (as in pie, cake, bread), sweet potatoes, dairy products (powdered or evaporated milk as ingredient in cookies, cakes, muffins, pancakes, mashed potatoes), butter
Vitamin E	Vegetable oil, margarine, dairy products, poultry, meat, fish, wheat germ (as ingredient in batters, meatloaf, sauces)
Vitamin D	Dairy products (fish oil for vegetarian and macrobiotic children)
Vitamin K	50% Made by intestinal bacteria; lettuce, broccoli, meat, cheese, butter
Vitamin B_1 (thiamin)	Fortified cold cereal, hot cereal, enriched flour and flour products, enriched pasta, meat, peanuts, sunflower seeds, peas, baked beans, chili with beans, peanut butter
Vitamin B_2 (riboflavin)	Milk, cheese, yogurt, cottage cheese, cocoa, watermelon, eggs, meat
Vitamin B_3 (niacin)	Enriched flour products and pasta, peas, potatoes, corn, peanuts, peanut butter; animal protein in foods like meat, fish, dairy products, and poultry supply tryptophan which body makes into niacin
Vitamin B_6 (pyridoxal phosphate)	Peanuts, peanut butter, bananas, corn flakes, potatoes, raisins, rice (rice pudding), chicken, wheat germ
Folic acid	Peanuts, peanut butter, lettuce (the dark leafy kind like Romaine), broccoli, whole wheat bread, fortified breakfast cereals, peas, wheat germ, spinach (if eaten)
Vitamin B_{12}	Meat, fish, dairy products, eggs. Only strict vegetarians and macrobiotics have difficulty in obtaining enough
Vitamin C (ascorbic acid)	Citrus fruits and juices, watermelon, tomatoes, strawberries, potatoes, green peppers, cabbage
Calcium	Dairy products are most common source; dark green leafy vegetables such as kale, swiss chard, and mustard, turnip and dandelion greens, and collards are also good sources but must be eaten first
Zinc	Meat, shellfish (probably not eaten too much by this age group), nuts, cheese, tunafish, garlic, chocolate, oatmeal (and soups and sauces made with meat)
Iron	Red meat, organ meats, liver, best sources; beans, chick peas, lentils, soybeans, pumpkin seeds, eggs
Iodine	Salt
Potassium	Fruits and vegetables (bananas and potatoes are good sources)
Fluorine	Water, some vitamin and mineral supplements
Magnesium	Vegetables, milk
Other minerals	Whole grain products (cereals, whole wheat bread) Wheat germ, vegetables, and fruits

your reluctance to prepare vegetables because your own mother ᴜᴠᴇᴦcooked them (stir-fry or steam them and season them); find some way of preparing liver without gagging; start eating fish, rice, buckwheat groats, eggplant, wholewheat bread, sweet potatoes, squash, and yogurt, even if you grew up in a family that lived on bologna sandwiches on white bread and meatloaf and mashed potatoes.

6. Do not be discouraged. Every day is a new eating experience, and one day your own child may actually say, "Please pass the spinach."

REFERENCES

1. Drummond, J.C., and Wilbraham, A. (1964): *The Englishman's Food: A History of Five Centuries of English Diet.* Jonathan Cape, London.
2. Dickens, C. (1839): *Nicholas Nickleby.* Chapman & Hall, London.
3. Anonymous (1975): *Nutrition Surveillance.* Center for Disease Control, Atlanta, Ga.
4. Shurtleff, W., and Aoyogi, A. (1975): *The Book of Tofu.* Autumn Press, Brookline, Mass.
5. Goodhart, R., and Shils, M. (1973) *Modern Nutrition in Health and Disease,* 5th ed., Lea & Febiger, Philadelphia.
6. Tappel, A. (1976): Vitamin E. *Nutr. Today,* July-August:4-12.
7. Chow, T.K., and Tappel, A.L. (1972): *An enzymatic protective mechanism against lipid peroxidation damage to lungs of exposed rats. Lipids,* 7:518.
8. Guthrie, H. (1977): Effect of a flavored milk option in a school lunch program. *J. Am. Diet. Assoc.,* 71:35–40.
9. Bettman, O. (1974): *The Good Old Days—They Were Terrible.* Random House, New York.
10. McBean L., and Speckmann, E. (1974): A recognition of the interrelationship of calcium with various dietary components. *Am J. Clin. Nutr.* 27:603–609.
11. Hambridge, K., Walravens, P., Brown, R., Webster, J., White, S., Anthony, M., and Roth, M. (1976): Zinc nutrition of preschool children in the Denver Head Start Program. *Am. J. Clin. Nutr.* 29:734–738.
12. Rozin, P. (1975): Psychobiological and cultural determinants of food choice. In: *Appetite and Food Intake,* edited by T. Silverstone. Dahlem Konferenzem, Abakon Verlagsgesellschaft, Berlin.
13. Tanner, J.M., Whitehouse, R.H., and Takishi, M. (1966): Standards from birth to maturity for height, weight, height velocity and weight velocity: British children 1965. *Arch. Dis. Child.,* 41:454–471; and 613–635.
14. Beal, V. (1961): Intake of individuals followed through infancy and childhood. *Am. J. Public Health,* 51:1109.

8 EATING TO GROW OLDER: Nutrition During Older Age

The nutritional needs of the older adult are similar to those of the younger adult. Unlike the younger adult, however, the older individual often cannot satisfy these nutritional needs without great difficulty. Many elderly individuals in this country are unable or unwilling to purchase or prepare a variety of food. They tend to follow simple and monotonous diets that are compatible with the physical, economic, and social limitations of their environment; unfortunately, such diets are often incompatible with their nutritional needs.

Discussing the nutritional needs of the older adult is simple. Ensuring that these needs are satisfied is not. An adult, regardless of age, makes nutritionally adequate food choices only if the foods are also compatible with his eating and life style. For example, turkey may be an inexpensive way of obtaining low-fat, low-cholesterol meat, but a woman of 83 will not lug home a 12-pound turkey for her solitary dinners regardless of its price. If prepared as suggested by a government-published cookbook for older citizens (1), spinach soup can be an excellent source of several nutrients; nevertheless, a recent widower who can barely boil water is not going to chop, dice, boil, and stir the seven or so listed ingredients. It is easier for him to make a cup of dehydrated soup, which requires only boiling water. Hence it is unrealistic to discuss the nutritional needs of this age group without also presenting the economic, physical, social, and psychological factors that affect the success with which these needs are met. This chapter does both.

NUMBERS

The elderly are increasing in absolute number as well as in their proportionate contribution to the population. Should the trend toward small families or childless marriages continue, the elderly may comprise one-fourth of the population by the year 2000 (2). The change in the number of elderly persons in our population must be most obvious to the elderly themselves: when they were young, around the turn of the century, the elderly made up only 4% of the population (about three million people). Approximately a thousand people reach the age of 65 each day, and, because of increasing longevity (particularly among women), many will eventually augment the numbers of those who are over 70 and even 80. In 1975 half of the older people in this country were over 73, and one million people were over 85; in the 1970 census 106,441 people were over 100 (2). In fact, the age spread among the elderly is so great that to call everyone over 65 old is as incorrect as to consider everyone under 21 a child. Indeed "old" is a relative term. To someone who is 69, a person of 76 is old; to the individual who reaches age 81, a person of 93 is old.

The nutritional problems discussed in the chapter do not develop at any particular age nor are they necessarily more severe among the "more old" than the "less old" of this population. There are individuals whose lifestyles and food choices at age 50 resemble those of an 80-year-old, and others whose appetite and digestive capacities at 90 would make a teenager blush. In 1975, 81% of those over 65 were fully ambulatory, and only 5% of the elderly are, at any time, in nursing homes, chronic disease hospitals, or other health care institutions. Hence the majority of people in this subgroup termed the older adult are "free living;" that is, they are not in any type of institutionalized setting. Moreover, they all have nutritional needs, and some have problems meeting these needs. Should this chapter provide some solutions to these problems, their capacity to continue to live independently and grow older will be enhanced

> The doctor examined the 83-year-old woman and said, "Some things not even modern medicine can cure....I can't make you any younger, you know."
> "Who asked you to make me younger?" retorted the woman. "I want you to make me older." (3)

NUTRIENT NEEDS AND THE PROBLEMS ASSOCIATED WITH MEETING THEM

Calories

The calorie needs of individuals decrease with age. Table 1 shows the recommended daily caloric allowance for those over 51 (the age at which old age commences according to the committee compiling the charts). Calorie needs drop below levels set for adults between 23 and 51 years of age. This decrease (300 fewer calories for men and 200 for women) is derived from studies on the reduced metabolic and physical demand for calories that characterizes those over 50.

> The basal metabolic rate describes the amount of energy needed by the body for its basic functions—e.g., the work of the cell in maintaining itself; the production of enzymes, hormones, and antibodies; the synthesis of new cells, such as red blood cells; the elimination of waste products through the kidneys; the maintenance of posture; respiration. This work is carried out by something called the lean body mass (LBM). The LBM is composed of muscles and organs such as the heart, liver, kidneys, skin, blood, and lungs. The fat cells, which contain their own supply of energy (fat), are not calculated into the basic metabolic energy needs of the body.
> As we age, the ratio of LBM to fat mass decreases. This change occurs despite the number of diets we go on or the amount of exercise we do. It occurs sometimes without any overt change in body weight. Since the amount of energy needed for metabolic activity is based on the amount of LBM, the decrease in LBM brings with it a decrease in the amount of necessary calories.

Physical activity also changes with age, although its decline can start decades earlier than the metabolic changes. Certain factors in the lifestyle of the older

TABLE 1. *Recommended Daily Dietary Allowances for individuals over 51 years of age*[a]

Nutrient	Requirement for men	Requirement for women
Energy	2,400 cal	1,800 cal
Protein	56 g	46 g
Vitamin A[b]	1,000 RE or	800 RE or
	5,000 IU	4,000 IU
Vitamin D_2	—	—
Vitamin E	15 IU	12 IU
Ascorbic acid	70 mg	70 mg
Folacin (folic acid)	400 μg	400 μg
Niacin	16 mg	12 mg
Riboflavin	1.5 mg	1.1 mg
Thiamin	1.2 mg	1.0 mg
Vitamin B_6	2.0 mg	2.0 mg
Vitamin B_{12}	3.0 μg	3.0 μg
Calcium	800 mg	800 mg
Phosphorus	800 mg	800 mg
Iodine	110 μg	80 μg
Iron	10 mg	10 mg
Magnesium	350 mg	300 mg
Zinc	15 mg	15 mg

Cal = calories; g = grams; mg = milligrams; μg = micrograms.

[a]These recommendations are based on a man weighing 154 pounds who is 5 ft 9 inches tall and on a woman weighing 128 pounds who is 5 ft 5 inches tall.

[b]Vitamin A requirements are expressed in two ways: as RE (retinol equivalents) and as IU (international units).

adult may, however, contribute to this decline in physical activity. Retirement eliminates the need to leave the house every day; a reduction in the size of the family to one or two results in fewer household activities; a move to a location providing services that formerly required transportation produces less walking than before; and an increasing array of physical infirmities leads to a predictable loss of activity.

Even if a person is physically healthy, the fear of inadvertently damaging something often prevents him from trying any type of exercise. If an individual did not exercise regularly when younger, the desire to do so as an older adult will be inhibited by a fear that any new or unfamiliar movement might "move something out of joint." We all know that a painful stiffness often results from moving a rarely used muscle. We assume, however, that with time (and enough complaining) the pain and stiffness will leave. The elderly person often does not think of such aches as temporary, especially if waking up in the morning with a new pain or difficulty with some movement is an annoyingly familiar occurrence. These pains come without provocation, and many believe that exercise will only increase the number of aches and pains with which they contend daily.

Obesity, which often accompanies old age, can increase the difficulty of moving, bending over, getting into and out of chairs, and walking up and down steps. Moreover, the physical environment can obstruct one's ability to exercise.

Difficulty in walking on streets because of ice, snow, traffic, crime, and dogs tends to restrict the frequency with which the older individual leaves his home. Finally, it takes a certain amount of caring about oneself to exercise, since exercise per se is not an intrinsically pleasurable activity for many, young or old. Other problems are often far more pressing than lack of exercise: inadequate heat or food, crime, or loneliness. Exercise is a luxury that many individuals feel they can do without.

Eating too many calories is a common problem. According to tables of the Metropolitan Life Insurance Company (4), 68% of women and 57% of men between the ages of 60 and 69 are 10 to 20% above their best weight. If the weight gain occurs gradually, it may not be perceived. In a recent study on the health status of almost 800 elderly persons in the Boston area, one investigator asked the participants to tell him how much they thought they weighed before they were actually measured. Almost all underestimated their weights, sometimes by as much as 50 pounds.

Certain risks to health are associated with obesity at any age (5). They include elevated blood pressure (hypertension), respiratory difficulties, increased prevalence of "adult-onset" diabetes (the main therapy for this disease, which occurs during middle or late life, may be weight reduction), increased pain from bone and joint disease because of the need to bear so much weight, and an increase in the levels of triglycerides (fats) in the blood.

Reducing may be very difficult, however, because of the lifestyle adopted by many in this age group. Snacking is common and often takes the form of tea and cookies, doughnuts, crackers, toast, or muffins (not celery sticks or green pepper). Persons with these food habits rarely attempt to change them. Moreover, the idea of caloric restriction is not familiar to this group, primarily because many grew up before the concept of calories and calorie counting was well known. Indeed many of these adults spent most of their adult life worrying about how to acquire sufficient food for themselves and their families, not how to restrict it. For these reasons the suggestion of a low-calorie diet to those who would not know the caloric difference between sour cream and yogurt has about as much chance of success in getting them to lose weight as telling a teenage girl to clean her room.

The chance of a successful reducing plan is lessened if it entails drastic changes in eating habits. If a man has been eating boiled potatoes with sour cream every day for 82 years, he will not switch to cottage cheese and grapefruit slices. If the cause of the weight gain is to be found in an eating style adopted only in later life, however, a diet change may meet with less resistance. Snacking alone or with a friend often grows out of loneliness and boredom. Filling up on pastries and bread instead of a planned and cooked dinner may occur after an individual suddenly finds himself eating alone after decades of sharing a meal. It may simply be too painful to eat a traditional meal alone.

Because these eating habits are common within this age group, opportunities for discussing such problems might be an effective means for solving them. Group discussions about eating, solitary dining, and snacking, as well as information on calories and suggestions for weight loss, would allow people with similar problems to share them. In addition, as shown by the success of such national group weight reduction organizations as Weight Watchers, group discussions may result in a loss of weight and, as an additional benefit, a loss of loneliness. One setting for such a discussion group is the site of government-sponsored lunches, especially since time for recreational activities is usually available before or after the meal. Senior citizen groups, Golden Agers clubs, even a morning gathering at a local doughnut shop could be the setting for a sharing of problems about eating and weight loss (although in the last example the meeting may have to move to less vulnerable ground, such as a local library). Merely having one person care about the diet and health of another is usually sufficient to ensure adherence to some sort of weight reduction program. In a neighborhood where many older adults live, one person can sometimes be admonishing another to put less sugar in her tea or to avoid a dessert because "the doctor said she should lose weight." Since many in this population live in housing for the elderly, a buddy system could be initiated so that those on diets could enjoy their cottage cheese together or entertain each other during those long winter evenings when eating seems to be the only diversion available.

Increasing one's physical activity is perhaps the best way to produce weight loss or at least prevent further weight gain. Moreover, it is a good index of the general physical and mental health of the individual. A social worker who counsels the elderly always asks her clients on their first visit if they are "good walkers." Their answers provide some insight into their lifestyle and well-being.

The weather sometimes presents an obstacle to outdoor exercise (the winter of 1977 is an example), and alternative exercises that can be done indoors are necessary. Walking or dancing around the apartment or house to music on the radio or television is a pleasant way of gaining indoor exercise (dancing is always fun). Simple calisthenics are also valuable, especially if practiced daily. However, as mentioned already, some people consider opening a can with a manual opener exercise, and such persons hesitate to try any activity that might "put a strain on the heart or a muscle." Demonstrating the safe way to exercise at a luncheon or on television using peers as teachers could be an effective way to overcome resistance to the idea of indoor movement.

> The efficacy of exercise on health and longevity was strikingly demonstrated when I bumped into what I thought was a well-maintained woman of 75 coming out of a health food store. Thinking that she perhaps maintained her vigor with something she purchased in the store, I asked her why she stopped here. "For the cookies," she replied, and then added that they were delicious. I asked her whether she baked similar cookies at home, and she laughed and said, "At my age, I don't bother anymore." I, of course, asked what her age was. "Ninety-two," she answered proudly, and then went on to tell me that she exercised every morning for an hour and had been on television the previous year to demonstrate her exercises.

An activity meter was developed in Germany for use with convalescents, and it is currently used in this country by physicians treating persons for obesity.[1] Unlike a pedometer, which monitors only walking or running, the activity meter records *all* body movements. The sensitivity of the meter to movement can be decreased by adjusting a setting on its side. The dial is calibrated in days, and the object of an exercise program using this meter is to accomplish five units worth of activity per day. The lowest setting registers extremely light activity, such as swinging the arms or swaying from side to side, so that even the most sedentary older adult can move the dial by doing very simple movements. Hence such a device immediately rewards the initial efforts at exercise and is very useful for those who have been confined to a bed or chair. Moreover, it tells the voluntarily inactive individual just how inactive he really is. Unfortunately, these devices are now too costly to be of value on a widespread basis; should such a model ever be available in a less expensive form, it would be an effective way of increasing energy output for those with an excess of energy intake.

The protein needs of the older adult are similar to those of the younger population. However, some older individuals need to eat slightly larger amounts than are recommended in the charts (6). Moreover, protein needs increase during and immediately after an infectious disease such as flu (6). Older adults are often more susceptible to such diseases, and they may need more protein during such a period. It would be wise to add chicken to the chicken soup for the person recovering from the flu.

Excess protein should not be eaten, however, as it may put a strain on the kidneys. The body excretes the nitrogen portion of the protein that it cannot use. This process involves a conversion of the nitrogen to urea, which is then excreted through the kidneys. Kidney function decreases with age; therefore it may be difficult for these organs to contend daily with consumption of excess protein.

> A new fad has recently appeared among health food advocates: the eating of predigested protein (which tastes as bad as it sounds). The protein powder is to be eaten three times a day in addition to the normal amount of protein consumed in the diet. Although it is known that Americans tend to consume more protein than they need each day, advocates are promoting this powder as a guarantee of adequate protein intake. Should an older adult consider eating this mixture in addition to his normal diet, he should first consult a physician, lest the consumption of too much protein result in an unnecessary strain on the kidneys. [Eating predigested protein instead of regular food as a weight reduction method has caused over 40 deaths (6a). This type of diet *must* be done under the care of a physician (see Chapter 4).]

The type of protein-containing food eaten by the older adult is influenced, to a great extent, by his lifestyle. Many high-quality protein foods (e.g., meat, poultry, fish) are expensive and simply cannot be afforded by many in this age group. These foods and others (e.g., milk) may be too heavy to carry and hence not purchased unless the individual has help shopping. Many of these foods are too

---

[1]The activity meter can be purchased from Peter Lindner, The Lindner Clinic, 12132 Garfield Avenue, PO Box 2097, South Gate, California 90290

difficult to prepare to make them a useful source of protein. To someone who is partially blind or arthritic, peeling an eggshell from a boiled egg may be so difficult the effort is abandoned. Cottage cheese and yogurt are protein-containing foods that are compatible with the lifestyle of the older person; hard cheese is also a possibility, although some consider it constipating. These products are inexpensive and lightweight, and do not need preparation. Unfortunately, the number of foods with these qualifications is small, and many people obtain their only daily protein from the government-sponsored lunch program. On weekends, when the lunches are not served, this population may not eat any high-quality protein at all.

Sometimes meat and poultry are avoided because they are difficult to chew. As our dentists continually tell us, teeth can present problems in later life. Decayed teeth, gum disease, or even ill-fitting dentures[2] can make the simple act of chewing foods very unpleasant. Some older adults buy baby food because it does not have to be chewed. Actually, some baby foods are excellent sources of high-quality protein. The strained meats come in small jars and thus are easy to carry and sufficient for one serving. They are low in salt, which is important for those on a low-salt diet;[3] they do not require preparation except warming; and since there is no waste they are a good value. The only negative aspect of baby food is the name. Few of us would like to admit we were eating this type of food (or serving it to our guests, as one hostess did, claiming it was a newly discovered paté). If the manufacturers of such foods repackaged them in adult-type containers (without the picture of a smiling infant on the label) and renamed them as low-salt sandwich spread, veal paté, or cracker dip, these foods could be bought without embarassment. Indeed should the trend toward a decreasing birth rate continue, baby food manufacturers may be forced to look toward the elderly as a new market, and these foods, newly labeled, may appear in the adult sections of supermarkets.

Dairy products are probably the most edible and economical source of animal protein for the older adult. They are easy to chew, less expensive than meat or chicken, and easier to prepare. Although they do not have the iron content of meat, this nutrient can be found in other foods, as discussed below. If eggs are eaten frequently, there is risk of increasing cholesterol intake above levels recommended by a doctor (some feel that two eggs a day contain all the cholesterol you should eat). Egg substitutes might be an acceptable alternative, and they have the additional advantage of lacking a shell.

Milk should be considered a high-priority food by the older adult. It is a palatable form of protein, vitamins A and D, calcium, and riboflavin. Many older

---

[2]Sometimes dentures cease to fit properly as the wearer ages and loses muscle and fat around the jaw area. The dentures become uncomfortable; yet many elderly do not want to go to the trouble or expense of having them remade and so have considerable discomfort when they eat.

[3]People on a low-salt diet should check the labels for salt content; some of the products may contain more salt than is allowed on such diets.

persons do not drink milk because they dislike the taste, associate it with children, or have an intolerance for lactose. The problem of lactose intolerance can be avoided by eating other dairy products, e.g., yogurt or cottage cheese. Transporting milk from the market to the kitchen can be a problem: in a liquid form it is heavy, bulky, and hard to carry, and in powdered form it is often available only in quantities that are inappropriately large for the single eater. Evaporated milk, however, may be purchased in small cans and some powrdered milk products come in small serving sizes. Some stores also sell fresh milk in pint-size containers.

Milk can easily be integrated into the eating style of this age group. For example, milk can be substituted for cream in coffee or tea, added to instant mashed potatoes or canned soups (e.g., tomato soup or chowder), poured on cold or hot cereal, added to cocoa, or poured over bananas, applesauce, or a baked apple. Individuals who eat many of their meals in restaurants with limited menus should order milk with their meal rather than—or along with—coffee or tea.

> In a neighborhood populated by many older adults, a doughnut shop and a fast food restaurant are frequented by the residents. Breakfasts at the doughnut shop usually consist of a doughnut or muffin and tea or coffee. The local fast-food shop often provides the evening meals and weekend lunches. Both of these eating establishments serve some highly caloric foods with low nutrient content (jelly doughnuts, muffins, apple pie, "milk" shakes, carbonated beverages).
>
> If the elderly customers were to include milk in their meal, they would be adding protein, vitamins, and minerals to a breakfast of primarily carbohydrates or a dinner of only hamburger and tea.

Carbohydrates

Carbohydrates (crackers, cookies, pastries, doughnuts, bread, muffins) make up a large proportion of the total diet of many older adults. Not only are these foods relatively low in nutrient content, their overconsumption can lead to obesity and may potentiate the appearance of diabetes in a diabetes-prone individual. Moreover, the consumption of such foods decreases the likelihood of the person eating other foodstuffs that are higher in nutrients and lower in calories (e.g., fruits and vegetables).

The eating style of some older adults can be defined as frequent snacking on tea and a starchy food. (A scientist who studied the health status of older people said he consumed gallons of tea and pounds of cookies during the year he visited these people in their homes.) Hence any attempts to lower carbohydrate intake must be compatible with their entrenched eating habits. The older adult who enjoys this meal pattern (i.e., frequent snacks rather than a three-course dinner at 6 p.m.) is reluctant to give up this distraction against boredom, regardless of the nutritional arguments. Suggesting a snack of carrot sticks and sunflower seeds to a woman without teeth who has been dunking her hard cookie in tea for the last 15 years is doomed to failure. People do not easily turn away from food habits that are familiar and satisfying. In order to introduce foods of some nutritional value into the tea-and-carbohydrate habit, the suggested new foods should be similar to those being replaced.

Cold cereals are a good snack food and appropriate for a midmorning snack or a light supper. The fortified and high-fiber cereals are excellent sources of nutrients and roughage, respectively. Instant hot cereals that need only be stirred into boiling water are also good snack foods. They are often sweetened and flavored with cinnamon, apples, or brown sugar, and this snack-like quality may increase their acceptability. Although their nutrient content is not as high as the multivitamin and mineral-fortified cereals, they are nutritionally better than cookies or candy.

Those who work with the elderly occasionally note a tendency among older adults to prefer sweet foods. This strong taste preference must be considered when recommending nutritious foods for snacks. Perhaps this tendency arose from a prior rejection of spicy foods, which may have become associated with unpleasant digestive aftereffects or the inability of some older individuals to taste a food as sweet unless it contains substantial amounts of sugar. Several types of vitamin- and mineral-fortified foods that resemble cookies or candy bars are now available, e.g., diet bars, granola bars, and breakfast bars. To suggest these foods as snack alternatives may seem to be nutritional heresy since these foods, with the exception of diet bars, are rather high in sugar; they are certainly better, however, than the cupcakes or cookies they may replace. Other sweet-tasting, nutrient-containing foods accompany a cup of tea are frozen French toast, waffles, pancakes (all of which contain eggs and milk), prepared puddings and custards, ice cream and flavored yogurt, toast with cottage cheese and jelly, bran muffins, and oatmeal cookies.

Fruits, of course, make excellent snacks. However, as discussed later, many fruits are not easily digested by the older adult. Moreover, they tend to be expensive (even in season), bulky, heavy, resistant to toothless chewing, or hard to peel for someone with arthritic hands or failing eyesight. Fortunately, when fruits were invented, someone thought of a banana, which, with the exception of its bulky shape, overcomes all of the objections listed above and indeed is highly favored by the older individual.

Fat

Fat intake apparently decreases as we grow older. Elderly individuals often find fats hard to digest and therefore eliminate high-fat foods from their diets. They rarely eat fried foods, for example, and may avoid mayonnaise, eggs, butter, and cream because of digestive difficulties. Meat, which is another relatively high source of fat in the diet, is eaten less frequently by this age group than by the younger population. In addition, many believe cheese to be constipating, so it is also avoided, with the exception of the soft cheeses (e.g., cottage or farmer's cheese). In fact, the consumption of fat may be so low among some members of this age group that the intake of fat-soluble vitamins (A, E, and D) may be deficient. Fortunately, low-fat dairy products (e.g., low-fat milk, yogurt, cottage cheese) are fortified with vitamins A and D, and many cereal products contain these vitamins as well as vitamin E.

Minerals and Vitamins

The inadequate consumption of several vitamins and minerals is characteristic of the eating patterns of many older adults. It is easy to see why. Their food choices tend to be extremely limited in variety. It is common for an older person gradually to eliminate many foods from his diet because of expense, difficulty in preparation, or problems in digestion. The foods that remain comprise a monotonous and often nutritionally deficient diet.

> In a discount supermarket in a neighborhood of elderly people, the woman who works at the checkout counter noticed that "the old people buy the same things over and over; some bread, cheese, maybe milk, maybe a can of sardines, cookies, and sometimes bananas. The ones with some money buy vegetables but the others never do. Occasionally someone comes early in the morning and buys the bruised and soft fruit; it is inexpensive then. Otherwise never."

Her perceptions were confirmed by a social worker whose clients are predominantly older women. The social worker said that fresh or frozen vegetables are almost never bought, and that canned vegetables are bought only rarely. Sometimes, she said, a woman who has paid attention to her eating habits for years makes sure she eats vegetables every day and always has a salad with dinner; but most avoid vegetables and fruits. They just do not want to bother. She added that the only time these people ate fruits and vegetables was when they ate the hot lunches sponsored by the government, and she worried about those who were too frail to get to the lunch sites.

Older people avoid vegetables and fruits because they are expensive, difficult to carry home, come in portions too large for solitary eating, and require cooking. Many older people do not eat raw vegetables as they may be difficult to digest. Another reason these foods go uneaten may simply be that they never were an integral part of the diet. Few 70-year-old men who dined exclusively on meat and mashed potatoes for 50 years are willing to start eating cauliflower or prepare a fresh salad for themselves. Moreover, the women who cooked the mashed potatoes and meat for all those years are probably unwilling to cook differently once they are alone. In addition, those who eat alone, no matter what their age, tend to eat simply and to decrease the time spent in preparation and cleanup. Although heating some frozen vegetables or making a salad may not require great effort, it may be too much for those who pay little attention to what and when they eat.

The lack of fruits and vegetables in the diet can result in certain vitamin deficiencies. Obtaining enough vitamin C (ascorbic acid) depends on the consumption of citrus fruits, other fruits (e.g., strawberries, watermelon, nectarines), or vegetables (e.g., cabbage, spinach, kale, "greens," potatoes). A steady diet of tea, toast, and cottage cheese obviously can result in a vitamin C deficiency. Folic acid is another vitamin lacking in such a restricted diet. This age group does not eat many of the foods containing this vitamin, e.g., spinach and other dark green leafy vegetables (which few of any age eat), fresh asparagus, lettuce, peas. Indeed folic acid deficiency is one of the most common dietary deficiencies among older people.

Some relatively minor additions to even a restricted diet can easily eliminate both of these deficiencies. Bananas and baked potatoes are good sources of vitamin C and do not cause the digestive problems associated with citrus fruits and other vegetables. Moreover, potatoes, which have only about 90 calories each (or the equivalent of two cookies), also contain potassium and protein, and bananas provide the diet with vitamins A and B_6, potassium, zinc, and magnesium.

Folic acid can be supplied by liver, which also contains iron, vitamins A and B_6, and riboflavin. It is not eaten frequently by this age group, however, perhaps because it is difficult to buy in small quantities. Moreover, the appearance of liver can be rather disagreeable to those who are inexperienced cooks, such as a recent widower (hamburger looks infinitely more palatable in a raw state). Liver must be broiled by those who follow Jewish dietary laws; this procedure may be a problem for those whose back or joint problems make bending over difficult. The strained baby food version of liver is an excellent substitute for those who do not want to confront liver in its natural state. It comes in very small quantities, requires no preparation, and can be easily spread on crackers or mixed with fried onions (for those who like this version). Kosher baby food is also available. In fact, baby food is a much better source of liver than frozen chopped liver, which contains salt and added fat.

Peanuts and peanut butter also contain folic acid; however, many in the 70- to 90-year-old age bracket grew up before peanut butter sandwiches became an American staple, and this food may be too unfamiliar to be acceptable to them. The willingness to try new foods decreases with increasing age. ("Why should I try it now? I've lived this long without it!") Fortified breakfast cereals are usually acceptable, however, because such products have existed for almost a hundred years; they do provide folic acid as well as some of the other vitamins and minerals, discussed below, that may be absent from the diet of the older individual.

The diet of the elderly person can lack other essential nutrients because he does not have the money to buy the foods that supply them. For example, riboflavin, which is found in meats and dairy products, can be lacking in the diet of an individual who can seldom afford to buy these foods and who, for various reasons, does not participate in a government-sponsored lunch program. There are some elderly who qualify for but do not participate in programs designed to supply them with supplemental money or food because they consider such help charity. Moreover, these people often deny to those trying to help them that anything is wrong.

A 96-year-old woman who is almost totally blind and partially deaf lives by herself and refuses to accept the care of a homemaker, which a social worker has been trying to arrange for her. When the social worker calls her and asks what she is eating for dinner, the woman always says she is having lambchops or steak, despite the fact that she cannot afford to buy anything but the cheapest of breads and occasionally some cookies and orange juice. Moreover, she has too little sight to see the stove as more than a blur. She is also too fragile and does not see well enough to take public transportation to the local school where she could get a free lunch. Fortunately, the people in the neighborhood look out for her; sometimes they pay for her groceries and carry them home for her. A local ice cream and sandwich shop gives her free soup, crackers, and tea every day for lunch, and the local policeman checks on her when she does not appear for a few days. When asked, she claims that she manages just fine and eats three good meals a day.

The diets of older adults can produce thiamin deficiency because they do not include the fruits and vegetables containing this nutrient. It is also supplied, however, by grain and dairy products as well as meat; consequently, thiamin deficiencies are common only among those who have an extremely restricted diet or who drink heavily. The absorption of thiamin by the intestine is reduced in alcoholism, and heavy drinkers should increase their thiamin intake. Unfortunately, those factors that often lead the older person to start drinking excessively also cause a lack of interest in his health, appearance, and diet; people who drink heavily usually eat an inadequate amount of nourishing food. (One female alcoholic in her eighties lived on whiskey and lemon meringue pie until a social worker took over.) Moreover, the older adult who is a heavy drinker usually does not have enough money for both alcohol and food and consequently buys very little to eat.

The intake of vitamin B_6 (pyridoxine), like that of many other nutrients, depends on a varied diet. Fortunately, bananas contain vitamin B_6 as do meats (remember those strained baby foods), tunafish, and fortified breakfast cereals.

Obtaining enough vitamin D depends as much on the overall lifestyle of an older individual as on his eating habits. Sunlight is an indirect source of this vitamin (the ultraviolet part of the spectrum changes a compound in the skin to vitamin D). Obtaining enough of this vitamin should not be too difficult for those who retire to the sunbelt or go swimming outdoors every day of the year, such as a group of 60- to 90-year old men in Boston (the L-Street Brownies). However, for those individuals who rarely go outside, or who do so covered with coats, hats, gloves, scarves, and boots 300 days of the year, the supply of vitamin D must be obtained through the diet, not by exposure to sunlight. The best dietary source of vitamin D is milk and other dairy products fortified with vitamin D. For those who do not eat these foods and who do not go outside frequently, an alternative source of vitamin D is cod-liver oil.

A light bulb that simulates the spectrum of sunlight has been developed. In a scientific experiment, residents of a home for the elderly were exposed to light from these bulbs. The results indicated that calcium absorption (which depends on vitamin

D) was higher among these subjects than among those who were exposed to light from normal fluorescent bulbs (7). If housing for the elderly were equipped with this type of light source, those individuals who neither go outside nor eat dairy products would have an alternative means of obtaining vitamin D.

Vitamin E occurs in vegetable oil, margarines made with these oils, cereal products, and baked goods made with margarines or vegetable shortenings. Unless the diet of the older adult is literally tea and toast, it is unlikely that vitamin E intake is deficient. Although some older adults take this vitamin as a supplement in the belief that excess amounts slow the aging process, there is no evidence that vitamin E makes us age less rapidly or prolongs life.

Vitamin B_{12} and K deficiencies are rare in the healthy older person. Some medications increase the need for vitamin B_{12} (hypertensive drugs or drugs for Parkinson's disease) or reduce the intestinal synthesis of vitamin K (antibiotics or sulfa drugs) (5). In these circumstances dietary supplements are probably the best source of the vitamins and should be prescribed by a physician.

Calcium is a particulary important mineral in the diet of the elderly as persons in this age group may be encountering the effects of a long-term calcium deficiency in their diets. The body needs to receive calcium from the diet each day to replace the calcium lost from the bones. If the diet continues to supply less calcium than is lost from the body, a decrease in bone mass eventually results (5). The disease osteoporosis, which is considered a disease of aging, is characterized by a loss of minerals from the bones. Although the exact cause of this disease is unknown, a chronically insufficient intake of calcium may contribute to its development. One therapy for this disease and for bone loss among the aged in general has been to increase the dietary intake of calcium (5). A calcium-deficient diet is typical among adults of all ages, and although the reasons for avoiding foods containing calcium may differ the result is the same. Since the loss of bone can be halted at any age by increasing calcium intake it is important that acceptable means of increasing calcium consumption be developed that appeal to those in their third decade as well as those in their eighth.

The easiest way to increase calcium intake among those who avoid dairy products (and "greens") is to add dry milk solids to those foods that are eaten. This can easily be done with soups and cereals. These foods are promoted as fast snacks or light meals because they require little preparation or cleanup. Instant hot cereals and soups are now packaged in single serving quantities and require only boiling water for their preparation. Canned soups are as easy to prepare and, except for a pot to clean, do not entail additional work. (Indeed, if the soup is eaten out of the pot, canned soup is also a one-utensil meal.)

The dried milk content of canned soups is very low, even in those soups that might be expected to have a significant milk content, e.g., chowders and creamed soups. A random look at the calcium content of soups from a major soup company showed the following:

New England Clam Chowder	16 *mg calcium*	2% *of RDA*
Cream of Mushroom Soup	16	2
Cream of Chicken Soup	16	2
Cream of Celery Soup	32	4

The instant soup-in-a-cup varieties are no better in terms of calcium content. A look at the ingredients of such soups from two leading manufacturers revealed that the major ingredients were sugar, food starch, hydrolyzed vegetable protein, and flavoring. The dried milk solids were not present in amounts great enough to make them a significant source of calcium.

These foods are excellent vehicles for added milk solids, as are the dried instant cereals. With some clever advertising directed at the solitary eater who likes to avoid excessive food shopping, meal preparation, or cleanup, soups and cereals plus milk could become an effective and acceptable means of increasing calcium consumption.

Other items eaten by the older adult to which additional milk solids could be added are bread, cookies, crackers, muffins, frozen pancakes, waffles, French toast, cereal, meatloaf, stuffing, meat patties, eggnog, and milkshakes.

A few years ago, a catfood company began marketing a dried pellet coated with milk powder. If catfood can be coated with this important source of calcium, dried cereal granules could also.

Television can be used to increase the consumption of calcium-containing foods among the older population and indeed to improve the overall nutritional quality of their diets. Soap operas, for example, are watched routinely by many in this age group, and the characters in the stories can become quite real to the viewers. Scanning some of these programs reveals a repetitive activity, eating, that is enacted by those of all ages as the major story lines are carried forward. In fact I watched, hypnotized, as a grandmotherly woman fed an 8-month-old some lunch—and the baby actually ate the food! These eating situations are wonderful opportunities for setting up role models who impart nutritional information on what older adults should be eating. The following scenes are examples of what could be done:

Lunchtime. The widowed father visits the kitchen of the neighborhood grand-mother. She says, "Stay for lunch. I just made some fresh broccoli, and we can have it with some tuna salad." She then pours him a glass of low-fat milk and, in the middle of a discussion of the latest scandal at the hospital, mentions that Dr. X told her to drink at least two glasses of low-fat milk a day to keep her bones strong.

Midafternoon. The mother of a thrice-divorced doctor gets together with her sister to plot the destruction of the doctor's fourth marriage. The sister asks for some coffee. The mother says, "Why don't you have some yogurt instead? At our age, we should really eat more dairy products, and I have never liked drinking milk. Joe (Dr. X) says that yogurt or cottage cheese is as good. If only he knew as much about women as he does about nutrition...."

The intake of iron is affected by ways in which the food habits of the older adult change with age. Iron intake declines if previous sources of iron (e.g., red meat and liver) are eaten less frequently or eliminated entirely from the diet. Moreover, the presence or absence of certain other foods in the diet influences the absorption of iron from the intestine into the circulation; hence modifications in their consumption can also affect iron status. For example, vitamin C-containing foods enhance the absorption of iron, and the addition of meat to a meal containing iron from a plant food (e.g., oatmeal) increases the absorption of iron from the plant food. A recent study demonstrated how the total diet may affect iron status (9).

A large group of older adults was given a variety of iron-fortified foods to eat; after several months the group's iron status was compared to that of adults of similar age and health who were not eating the iron-fortified foods. Because both groups had shown moderately low levels of iron stores before the study began, the investigators expected only the group receiving the fortified foods to show any improvement. To their surprise, both groups had increased hemoglobin levels (a measure of the adequacy of iron intake).

The result was hard to explain, but a plausible explanation was that both groups consumed more fruits and vegetables during the study, thereby increasing their vitamin C consumption and causing the iron in their diets to be absorbed more efficiently. Since the study had started in the winter and terminated after the summer, it was reasonable to assume that the change in seasons had produced a change in the amount of fruits and vegetables eaten. (The other explanation was that the attention and general medical care received by all the subjects had an undefined but real effect on their health.)

Other minerals that may be insuffficient in the diet of the older adult are zinc, iodine, and potassium. The best source of zinc is meat, but cereals, breads, pastas, and dairy products are all good sources of this mineral. Iodine is easily supplied in the diets of those who use iodized salt. However, for those on a low- or no-salt diet, iodine may have to be obtained from a supplement. Potassium is found in a large variety of foods, and a deficiency of this mineral is unusual among the healthy. However, the limited variety of foods eaten by this population can result in a dietary deficiency (5). Fortunately, one dietary staple of this age group, the banana, is a good source of potassium, as are potatoes, meat, chicken, hamburgers, oranges, and dill pickles.

NUTRITION AND LIFESTYLE OF THE OLDER ADULT

Eating a poor diet is not a characteristic unique to the older individual. Adults of any age (and children and teenagers as well) can make food choices that are nutritionally inadequate. The difference, however, between the poor diets of the older adult and his younger counterparts is that the former often eats a poor diet because *he has no other choice.* As the previous section pointed out, the food choices of the older person are determined less by what he likes to eat than by the economic, social, and health factors that limit what he can eat. Let us look briefly at these influences on the food choices of the older adult.

Health

A decrease in physical strength occurs with advancing age. The decrease may be gradual and insignificant for many until quite late in life; however, among its many consequences is difficulty in the acquisition and preparation of food. A loss of physical strength makes many ordinary activities slow and arduous: walking up and down steps, getting into or out of buses, pulling a shopping cart, carrying bundles, bending down or reaching up to put groceries away. Loss of muscle coordination, arthritis or other bone or joint diseases, swollen legs, dizziness, and loss of balance are additional examples of the health problems affecting the older person, and these cause food preparation to be reduced to the simplest methods possible. The mere act of opening a can or standing by the stove to stir soup can be painful for someone with arthritic fingers or aching legs.

Partial blindness can exacerbate these and other difficulties. If the loss of vision occurs gradually, the individual may almost unconsciously learn to adapt to this disability by reducing the number of activities that require acute vision, and as a result the person may not seek professional help when it is needed. Food acquisition and preparation is reduced to the minimum; cooking usually stops entirely; and the same food items are bought over and over again as the individual has learned how to open those packages and use those foods without much sight. These people, along with those suffering from other physical problems, usually cannot take advantage of government lunch programs because they are physically unable to get to the sites where the meals are served. In addition to losing the nutritional advantages of eating such meals, they remain hidden from those who could offer them social services to make their life easier and healthier (e.g., homemaker service, medical care, home meal delivery).

Physical Environment

The physical environment influences the ease and frequency with which older adults can purchase food, get to the sites where government-funded meals are served, and even go to the bank to have their Social Security checks cashed. Climate can be critical in preventing these activities. Cold, ice, rain, snow, and strong winds make traveling difficult and even hazardous for the older individual. Snow drifts 2 feet or more, blocking the street from the sidewalk, can seem as formidable as Mount Everest to a woman of 82 who must scale them with a bag of groceries in her arms.

Street crime is so unfortunately common as to be almost a truism when the problems of the older adults are discussed. Its frequency creates terror for those who are aware of its possibility each time they venture to the bank or supermarket. Some may prefer slowly starving to death on saltines and tea behind a triple-locked door to risking broken ribs and a concussion on the street.

Traffic and inconsiderate drivers increase the hazards of traveling to the store for those whose rates of walking do not allow them to cross intersections as rapidly as traffic lights or impatient drivers permit. Having cars drive around you on both sides is an unpleasant and potentially dangerous experience, and yet even in neighborhoods with a high density of older citizens little provision is made for longer pedestrian lights or policemen to help these people cross highly trafficked intersections. Moreover, the decline in city population has stimulated a movement of supermarket chains to the suburbs and their closing in city neighborhoods. As a result, the people who are left, often the older adults, must travel further to purchase food. Public transportation in many cities is nonexistent or sporadic, and this problem increases the difficulty older people experience reaching food stores or banks. Some neighborhoods or towns have bus service to supermarkets, and in rural areas neighbors often provide these services when they can. Lack of transportation is a major problem for many older people; in addition to the difficulty it adds to food shopping, it lessens their ability to get to sites where hot meals are served.

The kitchen facilities available to the elderly affect the ease and efficiency with which they can prepare meals. People who live in poorly maintained buildings may not have working appliances in their kitchens. Those who rent a room in an apartment or rooming house are often restricted to cooking on a hot plate and keeping their perishable items on the window sill. Even those still living in a single home may find it difficult to cook or keep food cold. A house that had a modern kitchen 35 years ago may today not have a working stove or refrigerator. The cost of repairing or replacing these appliances is high, especially for those who are barely able to pay the ever-increasing property tax on their homes.

> We bought a house from a couple in their eighties who had lived in it for over 25 years. The stove did not work at all, the cabinets were so high that reaching them required standing on a stool, and the refrigerator door did not close completely. Since the couple spent most of the year in Florida or with their children, this lack of a working kitchen did not critically affect them. There must be many others, however, who cannot escape and must contend with a kitchen that no longer "works" every time they try to cook in it.

Psychological and Social Factors

Many older people live alone. They are widows, widowers, or individuals who have outlived their friends and relatives. Their siblings may have moved or died. Their children often do not live near them, and even if they do their lives are sometimes so filled with other responsibilities or obligations there is little room for constant attention to the parents. There is an old saying: "One father can support 10 children, but 10 children don't seem to be enough to support one father" (1). Their "aloneness" is heightened by the realization that the situation will not improve and indeed will probably intensify. (Many younger adults also live alone, but they have friends, relatives, and the expectation that their solitary state will not be permanent.)

Eating alone has a direct influence on food choice. The types of solitary eaters and their habits in obtaining meals vary, from the individual who makes a meal of several items, sets the table, sits down, and eats leisurely, to the person who eats nothing at home except some instant coffee or tea and buys all his meals in a restaurant. The former are more apt to be women who have either adapted to solitary living by continuing to prepare food as they did when cooking for a family or husband, or women who have been single all their lives and always made sure they ate a well-balanced meal. The ones eating away from home are likely to be men whose culinary needs were handled by their wives. Finding themselves alone and forced to worry about their meals, many resort to eating in restaurants and eat nothing at home.

> A friend has an 86-year-old grandfather who recently lost his second wife. His granddaughter claims that "he never liked his wife anyway, but she was a good cook." He has now learned how to boil water, and his granddaughter is trying to teach him how to shop for food and prepare breakfasts and suppers at home.
>
> In spite of her efforts, he eats lunch 5 days a week at a school that serves meals to the elderly. He eats his evening and weekend meals at a local cafeteria because he will make nothing for himself at home except instant coffee. Since the granddaughter lives in another city, she worries that if he is unable to leave the apartment because of illness or bad weather he will not eat at all; consequently she insists that he keep food in the apartment in case these events occur. Nevertheless, he continues to resist her attempts to teach him how to prepare even the simplest foods because he hopes to remarry and hence resolve his problem.

There are those who simply do not want to heed their nutritional needs; they are totally disinterested in eating and in every aspect of their health. These people are usually depressed and either unable or unwilling to adapt to the changes in their life that bad health, poverty or the loss of someone they love has brought about. Since eating is, in a basic sense, an affirmation of life, they are totally apathetic about what and when they eat or if they eat at all. This type of situation cannot be solved by nutritional information, home-delivered meals, or food stamps. It requires the intervention and support of people trained to handle the psychological component of the situation. The nutritional aspects are secondary in these situations.

SOME SOLUTIONS

Governmental Programs

In 1965 Congress passed the Older Americans Act, which created the Administration of Aging. Financed by funds appropriated in support of Title IV, the Research and Demonstration Title of the Act, 30 demonstration projects were developed to gather information on various approaches to meal delivery in congregate settings. In 1968 this program received an infusion of $2,000,000 annually, which expanded the program to 32 sites in 1971. The need for a government-sponsored nutrition intervention program for the elderly was exemplified by the Recommendations of the Panel on Aging of the 1969 White House Conference on Food, Nutrition, and Health. By 1971 the popularity of 'these small-scale Title IV nutrition programs was so overwhelming that every effort to discontinue them proved futile. By early 1972 the time was right for Public Law 92-258, which authorized the Nutrition Program for Older Americans, Title VII of the Older Americans Act, as amended. Since the appropriations bill funding the program was vetoed it was not until July 1973 that the first meals under this program were served. This legislation alloted funds to every state and territory to provide one "hot nutritionally balanced meal per day at least 5 days a week" to eligible participants and their spouses (10). Those eligible are individuals 60 years or older, and the sites for serving meals are to be close to populations of the elderly in special need of this program (low-income and minority groups). In small rural areas meals are to be served at different sites, food is to be prepared whenever possible, and all elderly in need of such a service, regardless of background, are to be allowed to participate (10). In addition, the legislation made a provision for the home delivery of meals on a short-term basis for participants who cannot leave their homes. Supportive services—transportation, recreation, medical attention, social service counseling, nutrition education—were also written into the program.

There is no cost for the meal, but participants may make a voluntary donation. No tests of income are given to determine eligibility for the meals. The nutritional content of the meals is equivalent to one-third of the RDA for people in this age group. A new method of menu planning was developed for this program to be used by state and local program nutritionists to ensure that minimum nutritional standards are met (11,12).

> Nine nutrients ("indicator nutrients") were selected to be used as a standard by which the nutritional quality of a menu could be judged. The concentration of these nutrients in individual foods was translated into a unit system. The same was done with the calorie and fat content of food. Ten units of a nutrient such as vitamin A is the equivalent of one-third the RDA of that nutrient for men and women over 60. (The higher nutrient requirement, whether for men or women, was selected as the requirement for both. The riboflavin requirement for men is higher than for women; thus the requirement for men was the RDA used for meal planning.) Each meal should contain at least 10 units of each of the indicator nutrients and no more than 10 units of fat or 12 units of calories. Table 2 contains a sample menu-planning form (11) and shows that some nutrients are present in higher quantities than one-third of the RDA; neither calories nor fat, however, exceeds the required amount.

The meals that are delivered are the same as those served at the meal sites. Sometimes an additional meal, consisting of a sandwich, fruit, and milk, is also packed so the recipient can have something available for supper as well.

The nutrient intake of participants in the meals program has been shown to be better than the nutrient intake of the older adult population in general, and studies have demonstrated that the largest proportion of nutrients in their daily food intakes was contributed by this meal (13). Moreover, the ancillary activities of this program provide opportunities for its members to socialize, partake of the community's recreational facilities, and essentially break out of the lonely and solitary lives many of them had followed before such programs existed. In addition, these activities have an indirect effect on their nutrient intake: As these

TABLE 2. Menu planning form

Date Served 9/15 to 9/19/75
Week 2 of cycle

Project location: Senior Citizens Center, Oregano, Oregon
Menu planner: Alice Allspice

Menu item	Volume	Weight	Cals	Fat	Prot	Vit. A	Vit. C	Thia	Ribo	Nia	Calc	Iron	Phos
Monday													
Beef pie	1 cup	276	4	4	9	17	5	4	5	13	3	7	4
Lettuce and tomato salad	½ cup	53	0	0	0	2	4	1	1	1	0	1	0
Italian dressing	1 Tbs	9	0	1	0	0	0	0	0	0	0	0	0
Plain roll	1 roll	52	2	1	2	0	0	3	3	4	1	2	2
Baked apple	1 apple	177	2	1	0	1	1	1	1	0	0	1	0
Milk beverage choice	½ pint	241	2	2	4	2	1	2	8	3	8	0	6
Fortified margarine (for roll)	1 tsp	4	0	1	0	1	0	0	0	0	0	0	0
Daily total			10	10	15	23	11	11	18	21	12	11	12
Tuesday													
Breaded fish cheeseburger with bun	1 sand.	144	5	6	9	4	1	4	6	10	7	4	10
French fried potato rounds	½ cup	59	2	2	1	0	6	2	1	4	0	2	2
Tomato catsup	2 Tbs	33	0	0	0	3	2	1	0	1	0	1	0
Dill pickle relish	2 Tbs	30	0	0	0	0	1	0	0	0	0	1	0
Fresh tomatoes	¼ cup	45	0	0	0	2	5	1	0	1	0	0	0
Cabbage slaw with vinegar dressing	½ cup	77	1	0	0	0	13	1	1	1	1	0	0
Peanut butter cake	2½X3¼	70	3	4	3	1	0	2	2	6	2	3	3
Peanut butter cream frosting	4 tsp	25	1	0	0	0	0	0	0	1	0	3	0
Tea	1 cup	222	0	0	0	0	0	0	0	0	0	0	0
Daily total			12	12	13	10	28	11	10	24	10	11	15

participants become more interested in opportunities open to them, their interest in their health and in eating increases.

Other nutritional programs are in either the experimental or planning stages. For example, a formulated food which consists of a milk-powder base with added nutrients that makes a milk-shake-like drink when added to water is being considered as an inexpensive supplement for those elderly people who have nutrient needs not currently met by the Title VII program. The powder contains enough nutrients to make it equivalent in nutrient content to a meal (a similar product has in fact been used for years for geriatric patients in hospitals and nursing homes). It would be a convenient and nutritionally acceptable food not only for those whose nutrient needs are difficult to meet but for anyone who has difficulty obtaining groceries because of bad weather or poor health.

> Food similar to that eaten by the astronauts was given to older adults in Houston for a 4-month period. Twenty-one different meals consisting primarily of freeze-dried food (which needs no refrigeration) were developed at NASA headquarters in Houston and distributed to older citizens in the area who were unable to get to the hot meal sites or who would need meals on weekends. Preparation required only the addition of hot water; and the reconstituted beef almondine, cottage cheese, and other dishes had the same flavor and texture of fresh food. A few foods were canned and required only heating. Because the response to the meals was so favorable, the commercial firm that developed the foods for NASA is now thinking of making them generally available.

Private Sources

Much of the help the older individual receives in solving problems, of eating or otherwise, comes from friends, neighbors, relatives, and offspring. Many of the older adults help each other, especially those who live in the same building or neighborhood. Often a woman who can still cook and bake makes extra food and distributes it to those who eat most of their meals in restaurants. If someone is sick, a neighbor often goes shopping for him and brings soup or other cooked food so there is something to eat in the house. Relatives are also extremely important in ensuring that an older person can manage to live on his own. Providing transportation to the supermarket, carrying heavy bundles, or dropping by with some cooked food or fresh fruit can be an enormous help to someone who may not be able to manage these tasks without great difficulty.

> A lively woman of 82 who was just retiring from her job as a bookkeeper said that she depended on her niece to take her to the supermarket every Saturday afternoon. Although this woman was capable of shopping for some perishable items every day or two, she relied on the Saturday shopping for her meat and produce because these items were too heavy and bulky to be carried the several blocks between the supermarket and her home.
>
> Another woman with a widowed father prepared a chicken, a roast, or some stew once a week and put single-portion servings of the food into plastic bags that could be sealed and frozen. Her father kept these in his freezer, and in the evening he would simply place a bag in boiling water for a few minutes and then pour the contents on a plate for his dinner.

COMMENT

As we have seen, the nutrient needs of the older adult do not differ significantly from individuals several decades younger. Moreover, the food choices that derive from solitary eating are often similar among these two populations. However, the older adults do have special problems in regard to their nutrient needs as they are living, in a sense, on a time bomb. Many will eventually face the problems of advancing years: loss of physical power; an erosion of economic solvency; the need to adjust to solitary eating; increasing difficulties in food acquisition, preparation, and even digestion; and, for some, the tragic consequences of living in changing neighborhoods, where leaving the apartment house for food may be as dangerous as a soldier leaving a foxhole in the middle of a battle.

Fortunately, the problems of the older adult are being given the attention they deserve, and proposals for expanding present nutrition programs are being developed and seriously considered. These solutions are in their infancy, and the needs still far exceed the solutions. New developments, such as increased cash benefits for the older adult, easier means of obtaining food stamps, an expanded system of meal delivery at home, and an increased participation in the on-site meal programs, are being developed or tried.

However, the solutions are not and should not be entirely the government's responsibility. We all know older people. An increased sensitivity by all of us would make a significant difference in the ease with which these people can carry out the activities necessary to allow them to live independently. A bit of help and kindness from each of us—helping an older person to read a label, carrying someone's groceries, taking food to someone living alone, or inviting that person to dinner—go a long way toward helping the older adult meet his nutritional needs.

REFERENCES

1. U.S. Department of Agriculture (1974): *Food Guide for Older Folks.* Home and Garden Bulletin No. 17 (Stock No. 0100-03321). Government Printing Office, Washington, D.C.
2. Butler, R. (1975): *Why Survive Being Old in America.* Harper & Row, New York.
3. Rosten, L. (1968): *The Joys of Yiddish.* McGraw-Hill, New York.
4. *Metropolitan Life Insurance Company Statistical Bulletin,* Vol. 41, p. 4. Metropolitan Life Insurance Company, New York, 1960.
5. Watkins D. (1973): Nutrition for those aging and the aged. In: *Nutrition in Health and Disease,* edited by R. Goodhart and M. Shils, pp. 681-710. Lea & Febiger, Philadelphia.
6. Young, V.R., Perera, D., Winterer, J., and Scrimshaw, N.S. (1976): Protein and amino acid requirements of the elderly. In: *Nutrition and Aging,* edited by M. Winick, pp. 77–118. Wiley, New York.
6a. Glick, N. (March 1978): Low-calorie protein diets. *FDA Consumer,* p. 7.
7. Wurtman, R.J. (1975): The effects of light on the human body. *Sci. Am.,* 233:68–77.
8. Church, C., and Church, H. (1975): *Food Values of Portions Commonly Used.* Lippincott, Philadelphia.
9. Gershoff, S., Brusis, O., Nino, H., and Huber, A. (1977): Studies of the elderly in Boston. I. The effect of iron fortification on moderately anemic people. *Am. J. Clin. Nutr.* 30:226–234.
10. Administration on Aging, HEW Office of Human Development (1975): *AoA Federal Focal Point for Action for Older Americans.* AoA Publication 75-20143. National Clearing House on Aging, Washington, D.C.

11. Harper, J., Frey, A., Jansen, G.R., Fallisk, L., and Shigetomi, C. (1975): *Guide: Nutrient Standard Method Menu Planning and Monitoring*. HEW Office of Human Development, Administration on Aging, Washington, D.C.
12. Harper, J.M., Jansen, G.R., Shigetomi, C.T., and Frey, A.L. (1976): Menu planning in the nutrition program for the elderly. J. Am. Diet. Assoc., 68:529–534.
13. Greger, J., and Sciscoe, B. (1977): Zinc nutriture of elderly participants in an urban feeding program. *J. Am. Diet. Assoc.,* 70:37–41.

Subject Index

A

Acidity agents as food additives, 67
Action for Children's Television, 182
Additives, food, *see* Food additive(s)
Adenosine triphosphate (ATP), 141
Adipocytes, 85
Administration of Aging, 204
Adolescence, nutrition during, 155-186
Adolescents as overeaters, 94-95
Adult obesity, 89-97
Adulthood, eating during, 14-56
Adults, recommended daily intakes
    for, 15
Alkalinity agents as food additives, 67
American Academy of Pediatrics, 78
American Fried, 97-98, 111
Amines, 74
Amino acids, sources of, 19-20, 59,
    118-119, 133
Anorexia nervosa, 86
Anticaking agents as food additives,
    67
Antioxidants
  as food additives, 67
  as preservatives, 68
Ascorbic acid, *see* Vitamin C
Aspartame as a substitute for saccha-
    rin, 73
Athletes
  dietary needs of, 31-32
  glycogen and, 32
  nutrition and, recommended read-
    ing on, 53
Atkins diet, 105-106
ATP (adenosine triphosphate), 141

B

Babies, small-weight-for-date, 119
Baby foods, *see also* Infant feeding;
    Weaning foods
  as a food source for the elderly, 193
  homemade versus commercial, 151-
    152
  protein-calorie relationships in, 150
Banting, William, 105
Basal metabolic rate, 161, 188
Bettman, Otto, 176
BHA (butylated hydroxyanisole), and
    BHT (butylated hydroxytoluene)
    as food additives, 74

Biotin, 54
Blackburn, Dr. George, 103
Bleaching agents as food additives, 67
Blood pressure, high, and salt intake, 37
Bottle feeding versus breast feeding, 144-145
Bread as a source of nutrients, 20-21
Breakfast
  contemporary family, 7-8
  improving nutritional intake and, 25-26
Breast feeding, *see* Infant feeding, breast
    feeding
Butylated hydroxyanisole (BHA) and hydro-
    xytoluene (BHT) as food additives, 74

C

Caffeine as a food additive, 76-77
Calcium
  children and, 176-177
  content of foods, 121
  effects of underconsumption of, 33-34
  the elderly and, 199
  pregnancy and, 120-122
  recommended daily intake
    for adults, 15
    at age 0 to 36 months, 139
    for children and adolescents, 158
    for the elderly, 189
    during lactation, 146
    in pregnancy, 115
  sources of, 19
  vitamin D and, 139
Caloric consumption and thiamin, 172
Calorie-controlled
  formulated foods as a form of under-
    eating, 104
  meal plans as a form of undereating,
    101-102
Calories
  children and, 159-163
  the elderly and, 188-194
  functions of, 83
  infant feeding and, 134
  pregnancy and, 117-118
Canned goods and "open code dating," 62
Carbohydrates
  the elderly and, 194-195
  infant feeding and, 136-138
  pregnancy and, 116
Carcinogenic food additives, 71-74
Carotene, 15
Carrageenan as a preservative, 68